Blood Sugar Stability

How Glucose Regulation, Insulin Feedback, Stress, Sleep, and Fasting Shape Metabolic Health

Nathan Reed

PERENNIAL PUBLISHING

Published by Perennial Publishing

Paperback ISBN: 978-1-971996-54-7
Hardcover ISBN: 978-1-971996-55-4
E-book ISBN: 978-1-971996-56-1

Contents

Blood Sugar as a Regulated Variable

Blood sugar is easy to notice because it can be measured, but measurement does not make it self-explanatory. A number can appear precise, immediate, and objective while still revealing only one surface point in a larger regulatory process. The value may be real, but the meaning of that value depends on the system that produced it.

This distinction matters because blood sugar is often treated as if visibility equals explanation. A reading appears, and the mind moves quickly toward interpretation. It may be assigned to a meal, a fasting interval, a stressful morning, a night of poor sleep, or an isolated moment of glucose movement. Each of those conditions may matter, but none of them automatically explains the entire pattern alone.

A single reading can be accurate and incomplete at the same time. It shows where glucose availability is at one moment, but it does not show how that moment was created. It does not reveal how much glucose recently entered circulation, how much was removed by tissues, how much was released internally, how insulin feedback was coordinating uptake, or how counter-regulatory signals were preserving availability. It does not show the full history of timing, stress load, sleep and recovery, fasting state, activity demand, baseline tendency, or prior regulatory effort.

Measurement captures location, not explanation. It can identify where the system was at a particular moment, but it cannot automatically reveal the path that led there. Blood sugar regulation is a sequence, not a snapshot. A value appears after signals have already been interpreted, fuel has already been supplied or withheld, tissues have already begun responding, and prior conditions have already shaped the available margin.

This is why the same number can mean different things in different contexts. A value that appears after food input does not belong to the same regulatory situation as the same value during fasting, stress, morning transition, or recovery from prior movement. The number may match, but the mechanism behind it may not. Interpretation requires the sequence, not only the point.

Blood sugar is commonly reduced to food because the sequence is easy to see. Food enters. Glucose rises. The visible response appears to explain itself. This interpretation is understandable because food is the most obvious input. Meals have boundaries. They are remembered. They can be named and placed in time. When blood sugar moves afterward, the connection feels direct.

Food input does matter. It introduces fuel into the system and can change glucose availability. The error is not recognizing food as relevant. The error is treating food as the whole system. Blood sugar does not only reflect what entered from the outside. It also reflects what tissues removed, what the liver released, what signals coordinated, what stress load demanded, what sleep and recovery allowed, what fasting state exposed, and what baseline tendency the system carried into the moment.

Blood sugar is also easily moralized. A rise can be treated as failure. A decline can be treated as success. A pattern can become attached to discipline, food virtue, body judgment, stress response, sleep quality, or personal control. This moral framing assigns character meaning to a regulatory output. It turns a signal into a verdict.

That framing is not useful for understanding the system. Blood sugar movement is not a character statement. It is not a measure of virtue, discipline, effort, or worth. It is a signal produced by regulation. It reflects fuel availability, supply, demand, uptake, release, signaling, recovery, and constraint. Moral language does not clarify those relationships. It obscures them.

Blood sugar reflects glucose availability in circulation, and availability must be managed. The system requires enough circulating fuel to support function across changing conditions, but availability also has to be coordinated so that glucose is used, stored, released, and cleared in relation to demand. The issue is not simply whether glucose is present. The issue is how availability is regulated.

This is why blood sugar should be understood as a regulated variable. A regulated variable is not a number left to drift passively. It is monitored, adjusted, and maintained through feedback. It can rise, decline, stabilize, rebound, or return because multiple systems are continuously responding to changing conditions.

Blood Sugar as a Regulated Variable is the central orientation of this book. Blood sugar moves because regulation is occurring. It is maintained through input, output, internal release, insulin feedback, counter-regulation, timing, and constraint. The system does not hold glucose at one fixed point. It organizes movement around working ranges that can shift with context and over time.

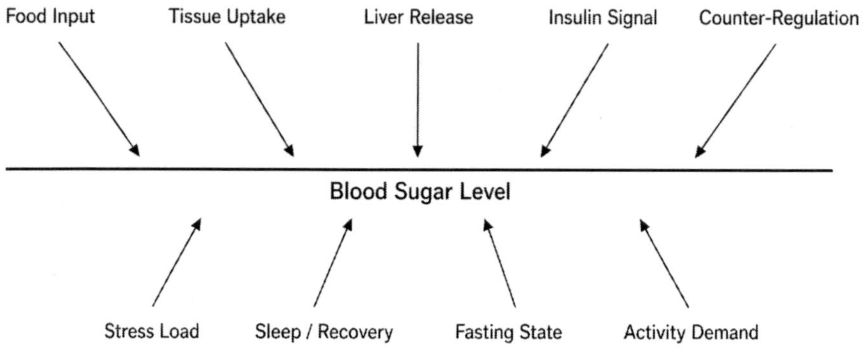

[Figure 1: Blood Sugar as a Regulated Variable]

The figure places blood sugar at the center because the visible number is the output being interpreted. Around it are the layers that help produce that output: food input, tissue uptake, liver release, insulin feedback, counter-regulation, stress load, sleep and recovery, fasting state, and activity demand. The purpose is to show that blood sugar patterns emerge from a system, not from one isolated cause.

The figure also prevents the model from becoming too narrow too early. If blood sugar is placed only next to food, then every pattern begins to look like a food response. If it is placed only next to insulin, then every pattern begins to look like a hormone response. If it is placed only next to stress, sleep, fasting, or activity, then each layer can become the whole explanation. The regulated-variable frame keeps those layers together.

This matters because blood sugar regulation is not a chain with one beginning and one ending. It is a feedback system. Food input, liver release, tissue uptake, insulin feedback, counter-regulation, stress load, sleep and recovery, fasting state, and activity demand continuously shape the conditions under which the next movement occurs.

Food input explains one supply path. Tissue uptake explains removal, use, and storage. Liver release explains how glucose can enter circulation from within the body. Insulin feedback helps coordinate uptake, storage, and reduced internal release. Counter-regulation helps preserve availability when supply needs support. Stress load can increase demand-oriented availability. Sleep and recovery shape timing, margin, and return. Fasting state shifts visibility toward internal control. Activity demand changes tissue output.

When these layers are viewed together, movement becomes less mysterious and less moralized. A rise after food may reflect incoming supply. A rise during fasting may reflect internal release. A morning rise may reflect transition from overnight regulation toward waking demand. A stress-related rise may reflect availability preservation. A decline may reflect tissue uptake and storage. A rebound may reflect counter-regulation after a prior correction.

Blood sugar is supposed to move. Movement after input, fasting, stress, activity demand, or morning transition can reflect regulation rather than failure. A system that never moved would not be adapting fuel availability to changing conditions. Stability is not stillness. It is movement that remains coordinated, contained, and recoverable.

Instability is different from movement. Instability appears when movement becomes excessive, prolonged, poorly matched, difficult to resolve, or repeatedly amplified. A rise is not automatically instability. A decline is not automatically success. A stable pattern has to be interpreted through timing, proportion, baseline tendency, recovery, and context.

A single reading therefore cannot carry the full meaning of blood sugar stability. It is one surface point. Stability is a time-based property involving patterns across minutes, hours, days, and repeated cycles. A number matters because it belongs to a sequence. It gains meaning from what came before it, what follows it, and what range the system tends to return toward.

Baseline tendency, variability, correction, return, and recovery all shape interpretation. A system may rise and return cleanly. It may appear calm while drifting upward over time. It may show repeated swings even when individual readings do not seem dramatic. It may correct one movement but overcorrect into another. The pattern over time matters because regulation is continuous.

Feedback is the structure that makes this regulation possible. The system senses changes in availability, coordinates signals, adjusts uptake or release, and reassesses the result. Insulin signaling, counter-regulatory signaling, tissue uptake, and internal release all participate in this feedback. They do not act as isolated forces. They function as parts of a control system.

A control system does not create stability by preventing all movement. It creates stability by detecting change, responding to change, and adjusting after the response. That distinction is essential. Blood sugar regulation depends on the ability to notice altered availability, coordinate an appropriate response, and then resolve that response when conditions change again.

This also explains why no single signal can define the whole system. Insulin feedback matters because uptake and storage must be coordinated. Counter-regulation matters because availability must be defended when supply is limited or demand increases. Internal release matters because food input is not continuous. Tissue uptake matters because availability has to become usable. Stability appears when these responses remain coordinated across time.

Correction is not failure. Correction is part of regulation. When glucose rises after input, the system must respond. When food is absent, the system must preserve availability. When stress signals demand, internal release may increase. When tissues remove glucose, supply must remain coordinated. Regulation is made of these adjustments.

Those adjustments also occur within limits. The system has regulatory margin, but that margin is not infinite. Chronic stress, disrupted sleep, aging, illness burden, low recovery capacity, reduced muscle buffer, repeated volatility, and elevated baseline tendency can narrow the space available for clean regulation. Under constraint, the same input or demand may produce larger, slower, or more effortful movement.

This book is not a diet plan, fasting plan, glucose-lowering manual, medical protocol, or optimization guide. It does not begin from the assumption that blood sugar is a target to force into a preferred shape. It does not treat food, fasting, stress, sleep, or activity as moral categories. It does not frame glucose movement as a score.

The purpose is interpretive. The book examines how blood sugar regulation works across food input, tissue output, liver release, insulin feedback, counter-regulation, fasting, stress, sleep, activity demand, recovery, variability, baseline tendency, correction, and constraint. Its focus is not what to do with a number, but how to understand the system that produced it.

That distinction shapes the entire book. The chapters that follow do not treat blood sugar as an isolated problem to solve. They examine the layers that make the visible pattern possible: regulation, feedback, baseline tendency, input, output, internal release, insulin coordination, counter-regulation, balance, overcorrection, baseline elevation, variability, fasting, stress, sleep, integration, constraint, and final interpretation.

The goal is not to make blood sugar seem simple. The goal is to make the complexity legible. Once the reader sees blood sugar as a regulated variable, individual patterns can be interpreted with less blame, less overreaction, and more attention to the system state beneath the number.

This orientation changes the reader's starting question. Instead of asking what one reading proves, the regulated-variable frame asks what processes may be interacting. Instead of treating movement as failure, it asks whether movement is coordinated and recoverable. Instead of isolating food, stress, sleep, fasting, or insulin as the entire explanation, it places each inside a broader system.

Blood sugar stability, in this frame, is coordinated fuel regulation over time. It is the system's ability to respond to input, preserve availability, remove glucose through tissues, release glucose internally, coordinate signals, recover after demand, and remain within workable patterns despite changing conditions. It is not judgment, perfection, or control of a single number.

Before blood sugar can be interpreted through spikes, crashes, targets, isolated readings, or daily variation, it has to be understood as a regulated variable. The book begins there, with the mechanism that makes blood sugar regulation possible in the first place.

The Regulation Mechanism

Blood sugar is often treated as a direct report on what was eaten. A meal raises it. Time lowers it. The reading is interpreted as a simple consequence of intake, a visible trace of recent food decisions. This explanation is familiar because it captures part of what can be observed. Glucose does rise after eating. It does tend to decline when food is absent. The pattern appears straightforward when reduced to these visible shifts.

The problem is not that this explanation is false. The problem is that it is incomplete in a way that distorts interpretation. When a partial explanation is treated as the full system, it begins to misrepresent how that system actually behaves. Blood sugar does not operate as a passive surface that food acts upon. It does not simply respond and then settle. It is being actively maintained, continuously adjusted, and constantly coordinated across multiple processes that extend beyond the moment of eating.

This becomes visible as soon as the pattern is examined more closely. Blood sugar can rise in the absence of food. It can remain elevated longer than expected after a meal. It can fall even when intake has occurred. The same meal can produce different responses on different days without any change in composition. Morning levels can shift before any food is introduced. Stress, sleep disruption, illness, prior activity, and the state of the system from the day before can all alter the pattern in ways that cannot be explained by food alone.

These observations are often treated as inconsistencies or anomalies. In reality, they are the visible result of a system that is regulating rather than reacting. Blood sugar is not simply being pushed up and down by external events. It is being actively maintained within a functional range by coordinated internal processes that are always operating, whether food is present or not.

This is the entry point of the chapter's central idea. The Regulation Mechanism describes blood sugar as a controlled variable. It is not a passive reflection of intake. It is something the body maintains through continuous adjustment because circulating glucose serves a critical role in supporting cellular function, and because excessive accumulation in circulation also requires management. The system does not wait for glucose to appear and then respond. It anticipates, adjusts, releases, clears, and redistributes fuel in order to maintain usable availability across changing conditions.

A controlled variable is not defined by its lack of movement. It is defined by the presence of mechanisms that keep it within a workable range despite variation in input and demand. Blood sugar moves, sometimes visibly and sometimes subtly, but that movement occurs within a system that is constantly working to prevent extremes, sustain access, and coordinate supply with use. Stability in this context does not mean flatness. It means the ability to move and return, to respond and recover, without the pattern becoming excessive, prolonged, or difficult to regulate.

Understanding blood sugar as a controlled variable requires expanding the frame beyond intake alone. Food contributes to blood sugar, but it does not determine blood sugar in isolation. The system is already regulating before a meal begins and continues regulating long after it has been absorbed. Incoming fuel is one influence among several interacting layers that shape how glucose behaves across time.

One of these layers is the movement of glucose into the system through food, where digestion and absorption introduce fuel into circulation. This input is visible and often emphasized because it is directly tied to eating events. However, it exists alongside a continuous process of glucose use.

Tissues draw from circulating glucose to meet energy demands, and this use can increase or decrease depending on activity, recovery needs, and broader physiological conditions. Clearance is not a passive process; it reflects active uptake and utilization that change as the system changes.

Alongside input and use, there is internal release. The body is capable of producing and releasing glucose from internal stores, particularly through the liver. This means that blood sugar can increase even in the absence of food. During fasting, between meals, or under certain stress conditions, internal release becomes a primary contributor to circulating glucose. The system is not dependent on external input to maintain availability. It has built-in mechanisms to sustain supply when input is reduced or absent.

These flows are coordinated through control signals, including insulin and a range of counter-regulatory hormones. These signals do not act in isolation. They function as part of a coordinated network that adjusts uptake, release, and storage in response to changing conditions. Insulin facilitates the movement of glucose into tissues and supports storage processes, while counter-regulatory signals can increase availability when needed. Together, they help maintain balance between supply and demand, preventing both scarcity and excess from becoming destabilizing.

Overlaying these processes are constraints. Sleep quality, stress load, illness, aging, recovery capacity, muscle mass, and metabolic flexibility all influence how effectively the system can regulate. These constraints do not turn regulation on or off. They shape how well it can operate. Under favorable conditions, coordination may be smooth and responsive. Under strain, the same system may become delayed, exaggerated, or less efficient in its adjustments.

When these layers are considered together, the idea that food alone explains blood sugar becomes insufficient. Food can raise blood sugar, but it does so within a system that is already active. The rise after a meal is not simply the result of intake. It reflects how input interacts with ongoing clearance, internal release, signaling coordination, and current constraints. The same input can produce different outcomes because the system receiving that input is not static.

This is why identical meals can lead to different blood sugar patterns on different days. The variation does not require a change in food to be explained. It can emerge from differences in prior activity, sleep, stress exposure, recovery state, or the timing of previous inputs. The system's starting position matters. Its capacity to coordinate matters. Its constraints at that moment matter. Food enters into this context rather than defining it.

Recognizing this does not diminish the role of food. It places it within a broader system where its effects are shaped by interaction rather than acting as a single cause. Input contributes to the pattern, but the pattern itself is produced by regulation. Blood sugar is not a direct output of eating. It is the visible result of how the system processes, distributes, and manages fuel across time.

This reframing also changes how stability is understood. If blood sugar is assumed to be a passive response, then stability is often interpreted as minimal movement. Fluctuation is seen as a problem to be eliminated, and flatness becomes the implicit goal. Within a regulatory system, this interpretation becomes misleading. Movement is not only expected but necessary. The system must be able to rise in response to input, provide fuel during activity, release glucose during fasting, and adjust as conditions change.

A stable system is not one that avoids change. It is one that manages change effectively. It can increase availability when needed and reduce it when appropriate. It can return toward its working range after a disturbance. It can handle variation without losing coordination. Instability, in this context, is not defined by the presence of movement but by the nature of that movement. Patterns become problematic when they are excessive in magnitude, prolonged in duration, poorly timed relative to demand, or difficult for the system to resolve.

This distinction becomes important when examining patterns that appear irregular. Blood sugar that remains elevated longer than expected, drops rapidly after a rise, or varies significantly across similar conditions is often interpreted as evidence that regulation has failed. A more accurate interpretation is that regulation is still occurring, but under strain or mismatch. The system is responding, but the response may be delayed, exaggerated, or constrained.

For example, if clearance is slower due to reduced tissue uptake or signaling inefficiency, blood sugar may remain elevated even after input has ended. If internal release is increased under stress, levels may rise without food. If signaling is mistimed, the system may overshoot or undershoot in its adjustments. None of these patterns indicate the absence of regulation. They reflect regulation operating under conditions that alter its effectiveness.

This perspective shifts instability from a binary state to a spectrum of regulatory performance. The system is always active. The question is how well its components are coordinating at a given time. When coordination is strong, patterns tend to be contained and recoverable. When coordination is strained, patterns may become more variable, less predictable, and slower to resolve. The behavior of blood sugar reflects this coordination rather than simply reporting intake.

Seeing blood sugar through this lens also clarifies why attempts to interpret isolated readings often fall short. A single number does not explain itself. It represents a moment within an ongoing process. Without context, it cannot reveal how the system arrived there or how it will adjust next. Interpretation requires attention to pattern, to the direction and duration of movement, and to the conditions surrounding that movement.

The Regulation Mechanism provides the structure for this interpretation. It frames blood sugar as something the body maintains through coordinated interaction between input, output, internal release, control signals, and constraints. Each of these elements contributes to the pattern, and each can shift depending on the state of the system. The visible result is not a simple cause-and-effect chain but a dynamic output produced by multiple interacting processes.

Once this framework is established, the next question becomes how the system organizes these adjustments. Regulation implies not only that changes occur, but that they occur in response to information. The body must detect changes in glucose availability, communicate that information, and coordinate appropriate responses across different tissues and processes. This requires a structure that can sense, respond, and adjust continuously.

That structure is built on feedback. Blood sugar stability depends on signals moving through loops that monitor change and guide response. The system detects deviations from its working range, initiates adjustments through signaling pathways, and modifies input, output, or release accordingly. These adjustments then feed back into the system, informing the next response. Regulation is not a single action but an ongoing cycle.

Understanding blood sugar as a regulated variable leads naturally into this next layer. If blood sugar is maintained rather than passively observed, then the mechanisms of maintenance become central. The Regulation Mechanism establishes that active control exists. The next step is to examine how that control is organized, how information moves through the system, and how coordinated adjustments are sustained over time.

The Feedback Loop Mechanism

Chapter 1 established that blood sugar is not a passive surface responding to food, but a controlled variable maintained within a functional range. Once that distinction is in place, the next question follows directly. If blood sugar is actively maintained, then maintenance requires a structure. Regulation does not occur without information, and information does not influence the system unless it is received, interpreted, and acted upon. The presence of control implies a process through which change is detected and adjustment is coordinated.

This is the role of feedback.

The Feedback Loop Mechanism describes how blood sugar regulation operates as a continuous cycle rather than a one-directional response. The system does not move from cause to effect and stop. It moves through repeated cycles of sensing, signaling, adjustment, and reassessment. Each change in glucose availability becomes information. That information produces a response. The result of that response becomes new information, which produces the next response. Stability is not produced by a single correction. It emerges from the continuity of these cycles.

Blood sugar regulation, viewed through this mechanism, is not linear. It is recursive. A linear interpretation suggests a sequence that begins and ends. Food enters, blood sugar rises, time passes, blood sugar falls, and the process concludes. A feedback interpretation does not have a fixed endpoint. Each stage feeds into the next. A rise in blood sugar is not simply followed by a fall. It initiates a series of adjustments that continue until the system moves toward its working range, and even then, monitoring and adjustment persist.

The loop begins with a change in glucose availability. This change may come from incoming fuel, internal release, or a shift in demand. Circulating glucose increases or decreases, and that shift is detected by the system. Detection does not occur in isolation. It is embedded in a network of signals that interpret not only the magnitude of change but also its context. The same numerical shift can carry different implications depending on what is happening in the system at that time.

Once change is detected, control signals coordinate a response. These signals influence how glucose is distributed, stored, released, or used. They adjust tissue uptake, modify internal release, and alter how fuel is allocated across the system. These adjustments are not static commands. They are proportional, conditional, and continuously updated as new information becomes available.

The response alters blood sugar again. Circulating glucose moves in response to uptake, storage, release, and use. This new state is not the end of the process. It becomes the next input into the loop. The system evaluates the result of its own response and continues adjusting if necessary. If blood sugar remains outside the working range, further adjustments are initiated. If it returns toward the range, responses may taper or shift. The loop continues regardless of whether input is present.

This cycle can be understood as a repeating sequence in which fuel enters or is released, glucose availability changes, signals coordinate a response, tissues adjust behavior, and the result feeds back into the system. The loop does not require external input to operate. It functions during feeding, fasting, sleep, activity, and stress. It is a continuous property of the system, not a temporary reaction to events.

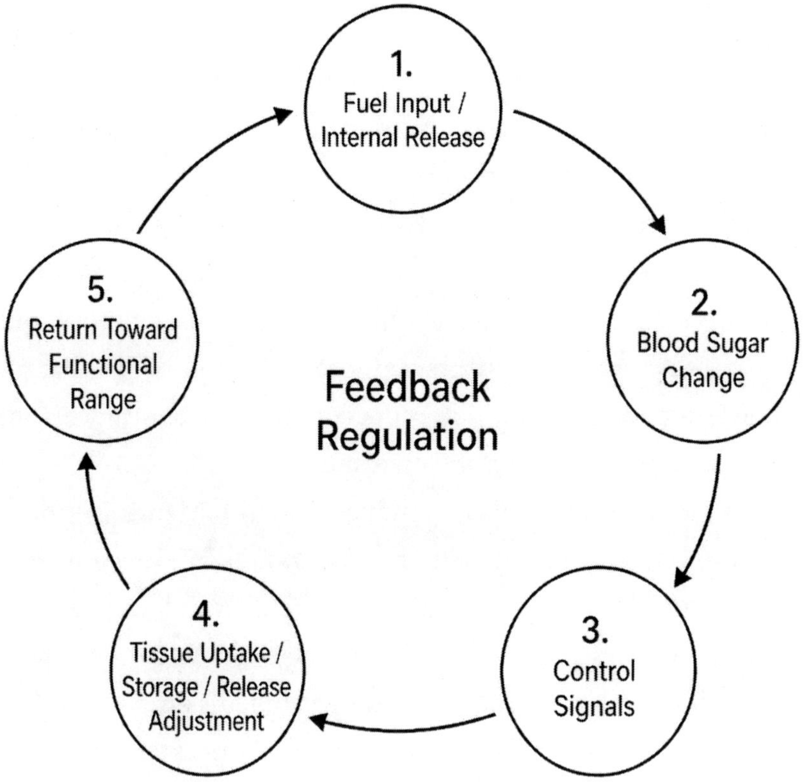

[Figure 2: The Feedback Loop Regulation Mechanism]

Once the loop is recognized, the distinction between linear and feedback interpretations becomes clearer. A linear model treats each event as isolated and self-contained. A meal is followed by a rise, and the rise is followed by a decline. The process is assumed to be complete once the initial change has resolved. A feedback model treats each stage as part of an ongoing cycle. The rise after a meal is not a discrete event. It is an input into a loop that is already active, and it modifies how that loop operates in subsequent cycles.

This difference becomes visible in patterns that do not align with a simple cause-and-effect chain. After food, glucose availability may increase, but the shape of that increase depends on how quickly tissues take up glucose, how much internal release continues or is suppressed, how signals coordinate uptake and storage, and what level of demand exists. The response is not determined by input alone. It is shaped by the interaction of input with the current state of the loop.

During fasting, the absence of food does not suspend regulation. The loop continues to operate through internal release and signaling adjustments that maintain availability. Blood sugar does not simply decline until it reaches zero. It is actively supported within a range that allows continued function. This support is not constant in magnitude. It adjusts based on demand, prior state, and constraints.

The feedback structure also introduces the importance of timing. A loop is not defined only by its components but by the coordination between them. Detection, signaling, uptake, release, and use must align in time for the system to maintain stability efficiently. When timing is well coordinated, adjustments occur in a way that contains variation and allows the system to return toward its working range without excessive oscillation.

When timing shifts, the loop can produce patterns that appear unstable. A delayed response can allow glucose to rise further before adjustment begins. An exaggerated response can reduce glucose more than necessary, requiring a secondary correction. Continued internal release after a rise can prolong elevation. Slower clearance can extend the duration of a response. These patterns do not indicate that the loop has stopped functioning. They indicate that the coordination within the loop has changed.

The Feedback Loop Mechanism makes it possible to interpret these patterns without reducing them to isolated causes. A prolonged elevation is not simply a result of input. It reflects how input, clearance, internal release, and signaling interacted across multiple cycles. A rapid decline is not a single overcorrection. It is the result of a sequence in which detection, signaling, and uptake combined in a way that shifted glucose availability quickly. Each pattern is a product of how the loop operated across time.

This perspective also clarifies that control signals do not respond to glucose in isolation. They respond to a context that includes demand, stress, sleep state, prior intake, and the condition of the system. A rise in glucose during physical activity may be handled differently than the same rise during rest because tissue demand alters how the loop prioritizes uptake and release. A similar rise under conditions of sleep disruption may produce a different pattern because signaling coordination is influenced by recovery state.

The loop therefore operates as a context-sensitive system. It does not apply a fixed response to a given input. It adjusts responses based on the interaction between current conditions and prior state. This is why identical inputs can produce different outcomes without requiring any inconsistency in the system itself. The loop is not inconsistent. It is responsive to variables that are often not visible at the level of a single reading.

Constraints shape how the loop operates without removing its structure. Stress, sleep disruption, illness, aging, reduced recovery capacity, and limited metabolic flexibility alter the efficiency and precision of feedback. Detection may become less sensitive or more variable. Signaling may become slower or more pronounced. Tissue uptake may be reduced or delayed. Internal release may persist longer than needed or respond more strongly to perceived demand.

Under these conditions, the loop remains active but requires more effort to maintain range. Adjustments may become larger, slower, or less coordinated. The system may need multiple cycles to achieve what previously required fewer. Patterns may become more variable, not because regulation has stopped, but because regulation is operating under constraint. The visible result is increased volatility, prolonged responses, or greater sensitivity to changes in input or demand.

This reinforces the idea that stability is not the absence of movement but the quality of movement across cycles. A stable loop does not eliminate variation. It manages variation in a way that remains contained and recoverable. An unstable loop does not lose its ability to respond. It produces responses that are less contained, less coordinated, or more difficult to resolve. The difference lies in how effectively the loop integrates information and adjusts across time.

The Feedback Loop Mechanism also clarifies why single adjustments do not define stability. A system may produce an appropriate initial response but require further adjustments to return toward its working range. The loop does not stop after the first correction. It continues to reassess and modify until the system stabilizes. This ongoing reassessment is what allows the system to adapt to changing conditions rather than relying on fixed responses.

Because the loop is continuous, there is no clear boundary between one response and the next. Each cycle overlaps with the previous and informs the next. Blood sugar at any given moment reflects not only the most recent input but the cumulative effect of multiple prior adjustments. The system carries forward information through its state, and that state shapes how it responds to new changes.

This continuity makes interpretation dependent on pattern rather than isolated events. A single rise or fall does not capture the behavior of the loop. The pattern across time reveals how sensing, signaling, uptake, release, and use are interacting. Stability is visible in the consistency of these interactions, not in the elimination of variation.

As the loop is examined more closely, it becomes clear that it does not operate around a fixed universal baseline. The range toward which the system adjusts is not constant across all conditions. It can shift based on long-term patterns, constraints, and adaptations. The loop maintains blood sugar relative to a working range, but that range itself is not static.

This introduces the next layer of the system. If feedback loops explain how blood sugar is adjusted, the question becomes what the system is adjusting toward. The concept of a stable range implies a reference point, but that reference point can change. The system does not operate around a single unchanging value. It operates around ranges that can shift over time as conditions and constraints evolve.

Understanding these shifts requires moving beyond the loop itself to examine how baselines and setpoints are established and modified. The Feedback Loop Mechanism explains how the system responds to change. The next step is to examine how the system defines the range within which those responses occur.

The Setpoint Mechanism

A system cannot regulate change unless change is compared against a range. A rise, fall, drift, or return only has meaning because the system has some operating zone around which response is organized. Without that orientation, movement would simply be movement. Regulation begins when movement is interpreted relative to a range that the system is working to preserve.

Blood sugar is often imagined as if the body were aiming at one exact number. In that view, every change appears as a departure from a perfect point, and every response appears as an attempt to restore that single value. This makes regulation seem narrower than it is. Blood sugar is not maintained at one fixed location. It is managed within a functional range that allows movement while preserving continuity of supply and control.

That range matters because blood sugar must remain available enough to support tissue function while also remaining regulated enough to avoid unmanaged accumulation in circulation. The system must allow glucose to rise when fuel enters, decline when tissues remove it, remain supported when food is absent, and shift when demand changes. Stability depends on coordinated movement around a range, not immobility at a point.

The Setpoint Mechanism explains this regulated baseline tendency. Setpoint does not mean a rigid number locked permanently into the system. It means the working range around which blood sugar response is currently organized. It is a tendency, not a fixed coordinate; an operating range, not a narrow target.

This working range is not random. It reflects the current state of the regulation system. It is shaped by what is entering circulation, what tissues are removing, what the liver is releasing, how control signals are coordinating those movements, and how constrained the system is. A baseline reading may appear simple from the outside, but it is produced by multiple interacting processes.

The setpoint concept becomes useful only when it is kept flexible. If it is treated as a fixed thermostat-like number, it loses the systems meaning. The body does not hold blood sugar at a perfect line. It organizes response around a range that can differ across people, shift across time, and change under repeated conditions. The range is regulated, but regulation does not make it permanent.

Baseline glucose can look like stillness from the outside. Before food enters, or during a quiet period when visible inputs are absent, the number may appear to represent a resting state. That appearance can make baseline seem like a blank starting point, as though nothing meaningful is happening until a meal, stressor, or activity demand enters the system.

Internally, baseline is active. Glucose may be released by the liver to maintain availability. Tissues may be drawing glucose from circulation for ongoing use. Some glucose may be stored, some may be cleared, and signaling systems may be adjusting the balance between release and uptake. Even when the surface appears quiet, the system is not inactive.

The liver is especially important to this interpretation because baseline glucose is not created only by recent food. When external input is absent, internal release helps maintain circulating availability. That release is not separate from regulation. It is one of the mechanisms through which the body prevents blood sugar from simply falling without support.

Tissue uptake forms the other side of the balance. Circulating glucose is constantly being removed and used according to tissue demand, signaling conditions, and the current capacity for clearance. Baseline reflects the relationship between release and removal. If release increases, uptake changes, or signaling coordination shifts, the apparent resting level can change even without an obvious external event.

This is why baseline is not the absence of regulation. It is regulation expressed as a resting tendency. The number visible during a baseline state reflects the balance the system is currently maintaining under its present constraints. Stress state, sleep state, recovery capacity, illness, prior activity, and repeated volatility can all influence whether that balance is steady, strained, flexible, or narrow.

Different people may regulate around different baseline tendencies because their systems are not identical. One person's baseline may reflect strong tissue uptake and lower internal release. Another person's may reflect greater liver output, different signaling sensitivity, lower muscle demand, or more accumulated constraint. The visible number compresses these differences into one value, but the value itself does not reveal the full system that produced it.

Liver release patterns can differ across individuals, and those patterns influence the range around which blood sugar is organized. A system that releases more glucose internally under certain conditions will tend to present a different baseline than one with lower release under the same visible circumstances. This difference is not simply about food intake. It reflects how internal supply is being managed.

Tissue uptake also varies. Muscle demand, activity history, recovery state, and metabolic flexibility all shape how readily glucose can be removed from circulation and put to use or stored. A system with higher tissue demand may organize glucose differently than one with reduced demand. The amount of glucose entering circulation matters, but so does the capacity and timing of removal.

Insulin sensitivity and counter-regulatory signaling add another layer. Control signals coordinate whether glucose is stored, used, released, or conserved. If the same signal produces different effects across different systems, baseline tendencies can differ even when visible inputs appear similar. Regulation depends not only on the presence of signals, but on how tissues interpret and respond to them.

Stress load, sleep quality, recovery capacity, age, illness, inflammation, prior volatility, and overall flexibility further shape the baseline. These influences do not rank people morally. They describe system conditions. Baseline glucose reflects internal organization, not character, discipline, or identity. It is a regulated output of the system's current structure and history.

The same person can also regulate around different baseline tendencies during different periods. Baseline is not frozen. It can shift as repeated conditions accumulate and as the system adapts to the environment it is repeatedly asked to manage. A person may show one pattern during periods of strong sleep and recovery and another during periods of sustained stress or low recovery capacity.

Sleep and recovery can influence the operating range because regulation depends on coordination. When recovery capacity is stronger, the system may maintain release, uptake, and signaling with less strain. When sleep is disrupted repeatedly, the morning baseline may reflect a different balance between internal release, stress signaling, and tissue responsiveness. The change does not need to be dramatic to matter. Small shifts in the resting tendency can alter how later responses unfold.

Sustained stress can also shift glucose availability. Stress-related signaling can increase the need to keep fuel accessible, even when food intake has not changed. In that setting, baseline may reflect a system preparing for demand or operating under strain. The result is not a simple failure of control. It is regulation organized around a different state.

Illness or inflammation may alter regulatory priorities. During periods of immune activity or physiological strain, the system may allocate resources differently and maintain glucose availability under conditions that do not resemble ordinary rest. Reduced activity can also alter the range by lowering tissue demand and changing the rate at which glucose is removed from circulation. Aging may narrow flexibility by changing recovery capacity, tissue responsiveness, and the margin available for adjustment.

Repeated volatility can gradually influence the usual starting state. When the system is frequently asked to absorb large shifts, recover from prolonged elevations, respond to stress signals, or compensate for inconsistent demand, the baseline tendency may drift. Baseline drift does not mean regulation has disappeared. It means regulation may be organizing around a changed working range.

Drift is best understood as a shift in operating state, not a collapse of regulation. The system still senses, signals, adjusts, releases, clears, and reassesses. But it may do so from a different range and with a different cost. More regulatory effort may be required to maintain continuity. Responses may become less flexible. The margin between ordinary movement and difficult recovery may narrow.

Starting state changes every response that follows. A meal, fasting interval, stress event, or activity demand never arrives into an empty system. It arrives into a system that already has a current operating range, a current level of constraint, and a current pattern of release and uptake. The visible response is shaped by what happens next, but also by where the system begins.

If baseline has shifted upward, a later rise may appear larger because it begins from a higher starting position. The input may be similar, but the response is occurring on a different platform. The rise is not only a property of what entered circulation. It is also a property of the baseline state that preceded it.

Recovery can also change when the starting state is constrained. A decline toward range may take longer if tissue uptake is reduced, internal release remains elevated, or signaling coordination is less precise. The system may still be regulating, but it may need more time or more adjustment cycles to return toward its working range.

A fasted reading may differ for the same reason. Food may be absent, but internal release and tissue uptake are still active. If the liver is releasing more glucose, tissues are removing less, or counter-regulatory signals are stronger, the fasted state may settle differently. The absence of input does not mean the absence of causes.

Stress responses also depend on the starting state. A stressor landing on a well-recovered system may produce a different glucose pattern than the same stressor landing after poor sleep or accumulated strain. The event is not interpreted by the body in isolation. It is filtered through the existing operating range and the system's available capacity for adjustment.

Setpoint does not mean flatness. A working range allows blood sugar to rise, decline, release, clear, and return while still being regulated. The presence of movement is not evidence against stability. Movement is part of regulation when it remains coordinated, proportionate, and recoverable.

The setpoint concept explains the range around which movement is organized, not the elimination of movement. A stable system is not one that never changes. It is one that can maintain coherence as conditions change. The working range gives those changes context.

Baseline glucose is therefore not a detached number. It is the visible surface of an active operating state. It reflects the balance between supply and removal, release and uptake, signaling and constraint, current demand and accumulated history. To understand the baseline, the forces that create it must be examined: what enters circulation, what tissues remove, what the liver releases, and how control signals coordinate those movements.

The Input Mechanism

Food is the most visible input into blood sugar regulation and therefore the easiest part to overinterpret. Meals have clear boundaries, identifiable content, and a memorable place in time. When blood sugar rises after eating, the sequence appears complete: something was consumed, and a response followed. Because the input is visible and the response can be measured, the connection between the two often feels sufficient as an explanation.

This visibility gives food a kind of explanatory dominance. It becomes the default cause because it is the most obvious event in the sequence. Other processes—internal release, tissue uptake, signaling coordination, recovery state—are less visible and therefore less likely to be included in the explanation. The result is a simplified model in which food is treated as the primary driver of blood sugar behavior.

That model is not entirely incorrect. Food does matter. It introduces fuel into the system, and that fuel can change glucose availability. The correction is not to remove food from the explanation, but to reposition it. Food is not the whole system. It is one component entering a system that is already active, already regulating, and already shaped by its current state.

The Input Mechanism defines this relationship. It describes food intake as an entry point into blood sugar regulation rather than as an isolated cause. A meal does not initiate regulation. It intersects with processes that are already maintaining glucose availability through release, uptake, storage, and signaling. The visible response after eating reflects how those processes receive and handle incoming fuel.

A system receiving input is never neutral. It has a current working range, a baseline tendency around which blood sugar is already being organized. It has a current level of tissue demand, a pattern of liver glucose release, a signaling environment influenced by insulin and counter-regulatory hormones, and a set of constraints shaped by stress, sleep, recovery, and prior activity. These conditions define the state into which food enters.

Because of this, the same meal does not produce the same outcome in every context. The food may be identical, but the system receiving it is not. The Input Mechanism explains why this variation is not inconsistency, but a reflection of changing system conditions. Input contributes to the pattern, but the pattern itself is created through interaction.

This distinction matters because input is easy to isolate while regulation is not. Food can be named, remembered, and placed on a timeline, but tissue uptake, liver output, signaling sensitivity, and recovery state are usually inferred only through their effects. The visible part of the sequence can therefore appear more causal than the hidden layers that shape it. Blood sugar regulation becomes easier to misunderstand when the most visible event is treated as the whole explanation.

The Input Mechanism corrects that imbalance by separating contribution from control. Food contributes material to the system, but it does not control the entire response once that material arrives. The system still determines how quickly fuel appears, how much remains in circulation, how much is removed, how internal release adjusts, and how long the movement takes to resolve. In that sense, food is not dismissed; it is placed in proportion.

Food must first become circulating availability before it can influence blood sugar. It is broken down, processed, and absorbed over time. Glucose does not appear all at once. It enters circulation at a rate that depends on digestion and absorption, creating a temporal pattern rather than a single event. The system responds to that pattern, not just to the total amount of incoming fuel.

The rate of appearance matters because regulation is time-dependent. A rapid increase in circulating glucose creates a different coordination demand than a gradual increase. The system must respond not only to how much glucose is present, but to how quickly it is changing. This introduces the need for coordination between appearance and response.

At the same time that glucose is entering circulation, it is also being removed. Tissues draw from circulating glucose for immediate use, storage, or future demand. This removal process operates continuously, influenced by tissue sensitivity, activity level, and signaling coordination. The visible blood sugar pattern reflects the balance between incoming fuel and ongoing clearance.

Control signals help organize this balance. Insulin signaling facilitates the movement of glucose into tissues and supports storage processes, while counter-regulatory signals maintain availability when needed. These signals do not operate in isolation from input. They respond to the presence of incoming fuel, the current baseline, and the system's overall demand.

Internal release adds another layer. The liver can contribute glucose to circulation even in the absence of food, maintaining availability during fasting or between meals. When food enters, internal release does not automatically stop. It may decrease, continue, or adjust depending on signaling and context. The visible response after eating therefore reflects both incoming and internally produced glucose.

Because these processes overlap, the same input can produce different patterns under different conditions. A meal consumed after strong sleep and recovery may enter a system with more coordinated signaling and a steadier baseline tendency. The response may be contained and recoverable, reflecting a system with sufficient capacity to manage the transition between availability and use.

The same meal after poor sleep may encounter a different environment. Stress signaling may be elevated, tissue responsiveness may be altered, and the baseline working range may be shifted. The incoming fuel is processed through these conditions, producing a pattern that reflects the system's current state rather than the food alone.

A meal after activity introduces yet another context. Activity can increase tissue demand and enhance glucose uptake. When food enters under these conditions, tissues may remove glucose more readily, shaping the visible response. The pattern reflects the relationship between input and demand rather than the input itself.

During stress, the system may already be maintaining higher glucose availability through internal release and signaling adjustments. A meal entering this state interacts with an existing pattern of availability. The response becomes a combination of incoming fuel and the system's effort to sustain readiness, rather than a simple addition of food.

A meal following a longer fasting interval may enter a system that has been regulating absence. Internal release may have been sustaining glucose availability, and tissues may have adapted to different fuel conditions. The incoming food modifies this ongoing state, producing a pattern that reflects both prior absence and current input.

A meal during low recovery capacity may require more regulatory effort. The system may still coordinate the response, but the process may be slower or less precise. Clearance may take longer, and the return toward the working range may require more adjustment cycles. The pattern reflects the system's effort to maintain stability under constraint.

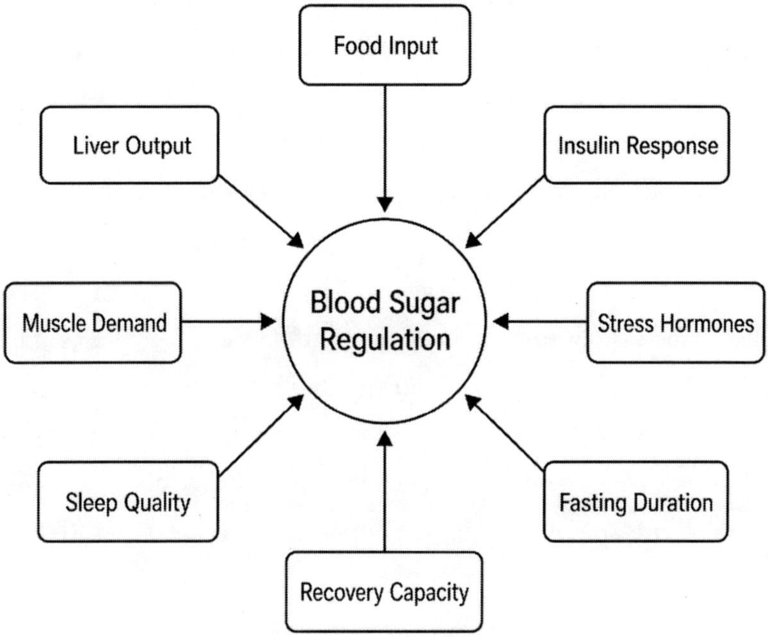

[Figure 3: Food Input Is Only One Layer]

Timing influences these outcomes because it changes the system state into which input arrives. A meal does not occur in isolation from prior conditions. It follows periods of availability, depletion, activity, rest, stress, and recovery. Each of these conditions shapes the baseline and the system's readiness to handle incoming fuel.

Timing is therefore not a rule to follow but a variable that modifies context. A meal consumed at different times may encounter different levels of tissue demand, different patterns of internal release, and different signaling environments. The resulting blood sugar pattern reflects these differences in state rather than the timing itself.

Food input also interacts with processes that are already active before eating begins. The liver may be releasing glucose to maintain baseline availability, and tissues may be removing glucose for ongoing function. These processes do not pause when food arrives. They continue, adjusting as needed to integrate incoming fuel.

The intersection between input and internal release is particularly important. Incoming glucose may coincide with ongoing release, creating a combined effect on circulating availability. Alternatively, internal release may decrease as incoming fuel becomes sufficient. The resulting pattern reflects how these processes are coordinated rather than the input alone.

Tissue uptake operates alongside these changes. Cells respond to signals that direct whether glucose is used immediately, stored, or conserved. The capacity for uptake depends on tissue demand, signaling sensitivity, and current constraints. This means that removal is not a passive consequence of input but an active part of the response.

Control signaling integrates these layers. Insulin and counter-regulatory signals coordinate the balance between input, release, and uptake. They help determine how glucose is distributed across tissues and how quickly it is cleared from circulation. The blood sugar pattern that follows reflects this coordination rather than a single directional change.

Food should not be interpreted as a moral category within this system. A blood sugar response is not a measure of discipline, virtue, or failure. It is a system output produced by the interaction between input and regulation. Attaching judgment to that output obscures the underlying processes that created it.

Food functions as both fuel and information. It introduces material that must be processed and integrated, and it signals the presence of incoming energy. The system responds to that information by adjusting release, uptake, and storage. The meaning of food lies in how it is handled, not in how it is judged.

The Input Mechanism places food within a broader regulatory context. Blood sugar behavior emerges from how incoming fuel interacts with tissue removal, internal release, control signals, and system constraints. No single layer defines the outcome on its own.

Understanding input in this way shifts interpretation from isolated events to system behavior. A meal becomes one moment within a continuous process, and its effects are shaped by what came before and what follows. The visible response reflects integration across time rather than a single cause.

Food input becomes meaningful through what the system does with it.

The Output Mechanism

Blood sugar is usually explained by what enters circulation, while less attention is given to what leaves it. Meals are visible, and the rise that follows is easy to connect to what was eaten. The decline that follows is often treated as a simple reversal, as if glucose fades away once the effect of input subsides. This emphasis on appearance creates an incomplete picture of regulation.

The asymmetry is not accidental. Input is observable and memorable, while output is largely hidden. Tissue uptake, cellular use, storage, and redistribution occur without direct visibility. Because these processes cannot be seen in the same way as eating, they are often excluded from interpretation. Blood sugar then appears to be driven primarily by what is added, rather than by the balance between addition and removal.

The Output Mechanism reframes this imbalance. Blood sugar output refers to glucose leaving circulation through active tissue handling. It is not waste, and it is not disappearance. It is movement into cells, where glucose is used for immediate work, stored for later, or redirected according to the system's needs. Every visible blood sugar level reflects both what has appeared in circulation and what has already been removed.

This dual movement changes the meaning of a blood sugar curve. A rise reflects the relationship between incoming availability and the system's current ability to remove it. A decline reflects the system's success in moving glucose out of circulation. The pattern is not a one-directional effect of input, but a continuous negotiation between appearance and clearance.

Output is therefore not a secondary event. It is a central component of regulation. Without removal, glucose would accumulate in circulation regardless of input. Without removal, the system would not be able to return toward its working range. Output provides the counterbalance that allows blood sugar to remain within a functional range across changing conditions.

The misunderstanding of output often comes from how declines are interpreted. When blood sugar falls after a rise, it is commonly described as the effect of time. The passage of time is assumed to bring levels down, as if the system gradually empties. This interpretation removes agency from the process and hides the work being done by tissues.

In reality, a decline represents active participation. Cells are drawing glucose from circulation, signals are coordinating uptake, and storage systems are capturing excess for later use. The visible reduction in circulating glucose is a result of these coordinated actions. Clearance is therefore an expression of activity rather than a passive fade.

Tissues are the primary drivers of this activity. Muscle, organs, and other cellular systems require fuel to function. Glucose is one of the fuels used to support that function. The demand for glucose is not constant; it shifts based on activity, recovery, baseline processes, and system state. This shifting demand shapes how much glucose is removed from circulation at any given moment.

Muscle demand is one contributor, but it is not the only one. Cellular activity continues regardless of visible movement. Organs maintain function, repair processes operate, and metabolic work continues across time. These processes draw from circulating glucose even in the absence of obvious activity, contributing to ongoing clearance.

This continuous demand means that output is always present. Even during fasting, when no new fuel is entering from food, tissues continue to remove glucose. The system must then balance this removal with internal release to maintain availability. Output does not depend on input to exist; it is an ongoing feature of regulation.

The idea of clearance becomes more precise when understood as movement into use and storage. Some glucose is taken up and immediately used to support cellular work. This immediate use reflects current demand and contributes to the maintenance of function. The removal of glucose from circulation in this case is directly tied to ongoing activity.

Other glucose is directed into storage. Storage allows the system to manage incoming availability without overwhelming circulation. It also preserves fuel for later use, providing a buffer between periods of input and periods of need. This buffering function is part of output because it removes glucose from circulation while maintaining access to it.

The distinction between use and storage is important because it shapes how output is interpreted. Immediate use reflects current demand, while storage reflects future demand. Both processes contribute to the reduction of circulating glucose, but they do so for different reasons. Understanding this distinction adds depth to the concept of clearance.

Demand plays a central role in determining how output unfolds. The same level of glucose availability can be handled differently depending on how much the system requires. When demand is higher, tissues may take up glucose more readily. When demand is lower, uptake may slow, and glucose may remain in circulation longer.

This variation means that output is not fixed. It adapts to system conditions. Activity state, recovery capacity, prior depletion, and baseline tendency all influence demand. A system that has recently used more fuel may respond differently to incoming glucose than one that has not. The visible pattern reflects these differences in context.

Recovery capacity also shapes output. A system with sufficient recovery may coordinate uptake and storage with less strain, allowing for smoother movement toward the working range. When recovery is limited, the same processes may require more effort or occur less efficiently. Output remains active, but its quality may change.

Insulin signaling is one of the coordinating elements in this process. It helps facilitate the movement of glucose into tissues and supports storage pathways. When glucose availability increases, insulin signaling adjusts to direct that availability into cells. This coordination allows the system to manage incoming fuel in a structured way.

However, signaling alone does not determine output. The effectiveness of a signal depends on how tissues respond to it. Tissue sensitivity, current demand, and system constraints all influence whether glucose is taken up efficiently or more slowly. Output is therefore shaped by the interaction between signals and tissue response, not by signals alone.

Counter-regulatory signals add another dimension. These signals help preserve glucose availability when needed, particularly during periods of low input or increased demand. By maintaining or increasing availability, they indirectly influence output by altering how much glucose remains in circulation versus how much is removed.

The balance between these signals contributes to the coordination of output. Insulin signaling encourages uptake and storage, while counter-regulatory signals support availability. The interaction between them helps maintain a functional range. Output reflects this balance as much as it reflects input.

The relationship between output and the working range is central to stability. After glucose appears in circulation, tissue uptake helps return levels toward the baseline tendency. When output is smooth and well-coordinated, this return can occur without excessive fluctuation. The system can absorb variation and reestablish balance.

When output is constrained, the pattern changes. Glucose may remain elevated for longer periods, or the system may require more time and effort to move toward the working range. These changes do not mean that output has stopped. They indicate that the system is working under different conditions, with altered capacity or coordination.

Constraints can arise from multiple sources. Reduced recovery capacity, stress load, disrupted sleep, altered signaling sensitivity, lower tissue demand, aging, or repeated volatility can all affect how output operates. These factors do not remove the mechanism, but they can change its effectiveness.

Under constraint, output may become slower, less flexible, or more effortful. Tissues may still remove glucose, but the process may require more time or stronger signaling. The visible result may include prolonged elevation or increased variability. The pattern reflects the system's attempt to maintain regulation under limitation.

Output does not operate in isolation. It is always interacting with input and internal release. Blood sugar at any moment reflects the balance between what has entered circulation, what is being added internally, and what is being removed by tissues. This balance defines the visible level.

A rise in blood sugar reflects not only incoming fuel but also the rate at which tissues are removing it. A decline reflects not only the absence of input but the presence of active uptake. A stable level reflects the equilibrium between these forces. Output is therefore essential to every pattern.

Understanding output shifts interpretation from surface observation to system behavior. Blood sugar is not simply a reflection of intake. It is a reflection of how the system is handling glucose across time. Output reveals the participation of tissues, the coordination of signals, and the influence of constraints.

The Output Mechanism connects directly to stability. Stable blood sugar depends not only on limiting appearance but on the system's ability to remove, use, store, and redistribute glucose in a coordinated way. Without effective output, input cannot be integrated into a stable pattern.

The strength of output is therefore not measured only by how quickly blood sugar declines. It is measured by how well tissue uptake, storage, use, and signaling remain coordinated as conditions change. A faster decline is not automatically better, and a slower decline is not automatically failure. The relevant question is whether the movement is proportionate to demand, recoverable within the working range, and integrated with the rest of the regulation system. Output is one side of that coordination, but it is never the only side.

Circulating glucose is shaped not only by what tissues remove, but also by what the body can release internally when external input is absent.

The Endogenous Release Mechanism

Blood sugar can change even when no food has been eaten. It can rise during the morning, remain stable overnight, or increase under stress without any recent intake. These patterns can appear inconsistent when blood sugar is interpreted only as a response to food. If food is assumed to be the only meaningful source of glucose, then changes without eating seem difficult to explain.

The Endogenous Release Mechanism resolves this confusion by introducing internal supply as part of regulation. Endogenous release refers to glucose entering circulation from within the body rather than from incoming food. The liver plays a central role in this process, acting as a source of glucose when external input is absent, delayed, or not aligned with current demand.

This internal release is not outside the system. It is part of the system. Blood sugar is not governed only by what enters from the outside. It is maintained through coordinated interaction between input, output, and internal supply. When glucose appears in circulation without eating, the source may be internal rather than external, but the process remains regulated.

Misunderstanding arises when blood sugar is treated as a direct readout of recent food intake. In that model, rising glucose without eating can seem like an anomaly. The assumption is that no input should mean no increase.

When the increase occurs anyway, it may be interpreted as a contradiction or an error in regulation.

The contradiction dissolves when internal release is recognized. A rise without food does not mean that nothing caused it. It means that the cause is not external. Glucose can be added to circulation by the body itself, using internal processes that maintain availability when needed.

This internal contribution becomes necessary because tissues do not stop requiring fuel between meals. Glucose is one of the substrates that supports ongoing cellular function. Organs continue working, metabolic processes continue, and the body maintains a baseline level of activity even in the absence of visible input. Blood sugar must therefore be preserved across gaps in intake.

This requirement changes the way absence should be interpreted. The absence of food is not the absence of regulation. Between meals, overnight, during extended intervals without intake, and during periods of increased demand, the system still has to preserve access to usable fuel. A narrow food-centered model treats these intervals as empty spaces between eating events. A regulation-centered model treats them as active periods in which availability must be maintained without relying on immediate external supply.

This is why internal release is not a backup mechanism in the casual sense of an emergency substitute. It is part of ordinary continuity. The body does not move from regulation to non-regulation when food is absent. It shifts the source of supply. External input becomes less dominant, tissue demand continues, and internal release becomes more important. Blood sugar stability depends on the ability to bridge those intervals without making availability entirely dependent on the timing of meals.

Dependence on recent food alone would create instability. Availability would rise after eating and fall during absence without a mechanism to maintain balance. The system avoids this instability by providing its own supply when needed. Internal release allows blood sugar to remain within a functional range even when external input is not present.

The liver functions as a central regulator in this process. It holds reserves and can generate glucose to support circulation. When signals indicate that glucose is needed, the liver releases it into the bloodstream. This release is not random. It is coordinated in response to demand, signaling, and system state.

Internal release and tissue uptake operate together. Tissues continuously remove glucose from circulation to support function. If removal continues while no food is entering, availability would decline without an internal source. The liver's release balances this removal, allowing circulation to maintain sufficient glucose.

This balance is dynamic rather than static. Tissue uptake may increase or decrease based on demand, and internal release adjusts accordingly. Blood sugar at any moment reflects the interaction between what is being removed and what is being supplied internally. Stability depends on coordination between these processes.

This coordination also prevents internal release from being misunderstood as the opposite of clearance. Tissue uptake and liver release are not competing in a simple sense, with one side trying to raise blood sugar and the other trying to lower it. They are paired processes within the same regulatory problem. Tissues remove glucose because function continues. The liver releases glucose because availability has to be preserved while that removal continues. The visible level reflects the relationship between these two movements.

When this relationship is well matched, blood sugar may appear steady even though a great deal is happening underneath. Tissues are drawing fuel, the liver is contributing supply, and signals are adjusting both sides of the exchange. Stability can therefore look quiet from the outside while the system remains active internally. The number may appear unchanged, but the unchanged number is the result of coordinated movement, not the absence of movement.

Fasting provides a clear context for this coordination. When food input is absent, the system does not stop regulating. It shifts emphasis toward internal mechanisms. The body relies more heavily on endogenous release to maintain glucose availability while tissues continue to draw from circulation.

During fasting, internal release becomes a primary contributor to blood sugar. This does not mean that regulation is reduced. It means that the source of glucose has changed. The system continues to maintain availability, but it does so using internal supply rather than external input.

Morning hours illustrate another form of this mechanism. The transition from sleep to wakefulness involves a shift in demand. The body prepares for activity, alertness, and engagement with the environment. Internal release can contribute to this preparation by increasing glucose availability in anticipation of need.

This increase is not a contradiction of regulation. It is an example of regulation anticipating demand. The system does not wait for food to arrive before making fuel available. It adjusts supply in advance, using internal release to support the transition into waking activity.

Stress introduces a similar dynamic. When the system perceives demand, whether physical or cognitive, it may increase glucose availability to support that demand. Internal release becomes a way of ensuring that fuel is accessible even if no food has been consumed.

This response is not a failure of control. It reflects the system's prioritization of availability. Stress signaling can influence how much glucose is released and how it is distributed. The resulting pattern may include rising blood sugar without eating, but this rise is aligned with perceived demand.

Sleep disruption can also influence endogenous release. Changes in sleep quality or duration can alter recovery state, signaling patterns, and the timing of internal processes. These changes may affect how the liver releases glucose and how the system maintains availability during the morning transition.

When sleep is disrupted, the coordination between release and uptake may shift. Internal release may be more pronounced or differently timed, and tissue responsiveness may also change. The visible result can be a different pattern of blood sugar despite similar external conditions.

Demand states extend beyond stress and activity. The body may require additional glucose during recovery processes, periods of illness-like demand, or shifts in metabolic activity. Internal release supports these needs by providing fuel when external input is not sufficient or not present.

The system does not treat all demand equally. It adjusts internal release based on context, balancing availability with conservation. This adjustment requires coordination between signals that promote release and signals that limit it. The goal is not maximal release but appropriate release.

Insulin signaling and counter-regulatory signals are part of this coordination. Insulin helps direct glucose into tissues and storage, while counter-regulatory signals support availability when needed. Endogenous release operates within this signaling environment, responding to cues that indicate whether glucose should be preserved or made available.

The balance between these signals influences how internal release contributes to blood sugar. If availability is needed, release may increase. If storage and uptake are prioritized, release may decrease. The pattern reflects coordination rather than a single directional force.

This is why endogenous release should not be interpreted as merely a glucose-raising event. It is a context-sensitive supply adjustment. In one state, internal release may preserve availability during absence. In another, it may support the transition into waking demand. In another, it may respond to stress signaling or increased functional need. The same mechanism can appear differently depending on the context that activates it.

The distinction matters because visible blood sugar movement alone does not reveal the reason for release. A rise in the morning, a rise during stress, and maintenance during fasting can all involve internal supply, but they are not identical events. Each belongs to a different regulatory situation. Understanding endogenous release means seeing the shared mechanism while still recognizing that the trigger, timing, and system state may differ.

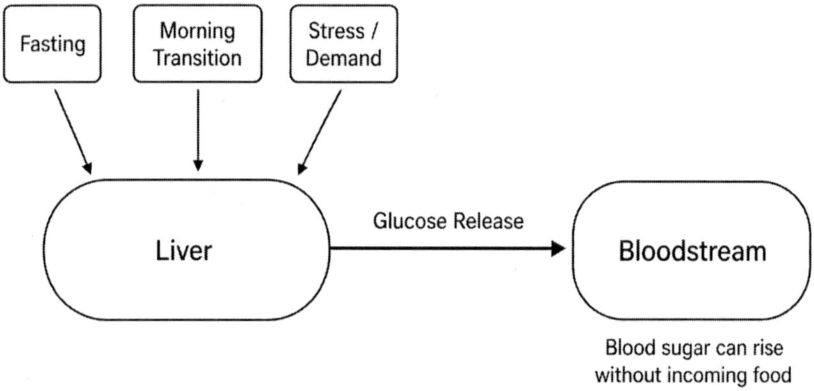

[Figure 4: Endogenous Release]

Because internal release is less visible than food input, it can be misread. Blood sugar rising without eating may be interpreted as random or problematic when the internal source is not considered. The pattern can appear disconnected from behavior, leading to confusion about what is driving the change.

Reframing internal release as part of regulation changes this interpretation. A rise without food becomes understandable as an internally generated adjustment rather than an unexplained event. Blood sugar is not simply responding to intake; it is being actively managed through multiple sources of supply.

This reframing also clarifies that regulation involves both maintaining availability and preventing excess. Internal release must be sufficient to support tissues but coordinated so that it does not produce prolonged elevation. The balance between release and uptake determines whether the system remains within its working range.

Constraints can influence this balance. Stress load, sleep disruption, recovery limitations, and prior conditions can alter how release is coordinated. The system may still regulate, but it may require more effort or produce patterns that are less stable or more variable.

Endogenous release therefore contributes to both stability and variability. When well-coordinated, it supports continuity of supply across time. When constrained, it can interact with other factors to produce patterns that require additional adjustment. The mechanism itself remains present, but its expression can change.

Blood sugar stability depends on the integration of input, output, and internal release. External fuel provides one source of glucose, tissue uptake removes and redistributes it, and internal release maintains availability when input is absent or insufficient. These processes operate together to sustain balance.

Circulating glucose is shaped by the combined effect of these layers. What enters from food, what is released internally, and what is removed by tissues all contribute to the visible level. Understanding this interaction provides a more complete view of blood sugar behavior.

Internal release highlights that regulation is continuous rather than event-based. The system does not wait for input to act. It anticipates, adjusts, and responds to maintain availability across changing conditions. Blood sugar reflects this ongoing coordination rather than isolated events.

The Endogenous Release Mechanism reveals that the body can supply glucose when needed, preserving function even in the absence of food. This capacity allows the system to remain stable across time, bridging gaps between input and supporting periods of increased demand.

At the same time, this mechanism requires coordination with signals that regulate when glucose should be added to circulation and when it should be removed. The balance between these signals determines how effectively internal release contributes to stability without creating excess.

The Insulin Regulation Mechanism

Insulin is often discussed as if it were a force acting on blood sugar, when it is better understood as a signal that coordinates regulation. The narrower interpretation treats insulin mainly as something that pushes glucose downward. In that view, glucose rises, insulin appears, and blood sugar is lowered. The sequence is recognizable, but it compresses the mechanism into one action and removes the broader regulatory context.

Insulin does help move glucose out of circulation, but that is not the same as saying insulin is merely a glucose-lowering force. It communicates information about fuel availability and helps tissues coordinate what should happen when that availability changes. A rise in glucose is not only a number to be reduced. It is a signal that incoming energy is present and must be distributed, used, stored, or balanced against internal release.

The Insulin Regulation Mechanism explains insulin as part of the communication layer of blood sugar regulation. Insulin helps align glucose availability with tissue uptake, storage, and metabolic direction. It supports the shift from preserving supply toward handling incoming fuel. This makes insulin a coordinating signal inside the larger system, not the entire system itself.

This distinction matters because insulin is often misunderstood in two opposing ways. It may be reduced to a simple blood sugar-lowering mechanism, or it may be treated as a problem signal. Both interpretations flatten its role. Insulin is not the enemy of metabolic stability. It is one of the signals through which stability is maintained.

A signal does not operate by force alone. It conveys information that tissues must interpret. Insulin tells the system that fuel is available and that uptake, storage, and reduced internal release may be appropriate. The effect of that signal depends on timing, tissue response, current demand, recovery capacity, stress load, sleep state, and the existing working range.

This means insulin presence does not explain the entire blood sugar pattern. A signal must be received by tissues capable of responding to it. If tissue demand is high, glucose may be taken up differently than when demand is low. If recovery capacity is constrained or stress signaling is elevated, the same insulin signal may produce a different regulatory pattern. Insulin operates within context.

The signal-versus-force distinction also changes how glucose movement is interpreted. When blood sugar declines after rising, insulin may be participating in the clearance process, but the decline is not caused by insulin acting alone. Tissues remove glucose, storage pathways accept fuel, liver release may be reduced, and demand conditions shape the rate of movement. Insulin helps coordinate those layers.

Tissue uptake is one of the clearest places where insulin's coordinating role becomes visible. When glucose availability rises, tissues need instruction about whether to receive, use, or store incoming fuel. Insulin helps facilitate this movement into tissues. It does not make uptake meaningful by itself; it helps align uptake with the presence of available fuel.

Glucose clearance therefore depends on both the signal and the tissue response. Insulin may indicate that glucose should move out of circulation, but tissues still determine how effectively that signal becomes action. Muscle demand, prior activity, baseline tendency, and recovery state all influence the capacity for uptake. The response is a relationship between signal and system state.

Storage is another part of insulin's regulatory role. When glucose availability exceeds immediate demand, some fuel can be stored for later access. Storage is not a moral category. It is part of how the body prevents circulating fuel from remaining unmanaged while preserving availability for future use. Insulin helps direct this transition from immediate circulation into reserve.

This storage function is often misunderstood because storage is frequently pulled into weight-centered or moralized interpretations. Within blood sugar regulation, storage is a stabilizing process. It moves glucose out of circulation, reduces immediate pressure on the bloodstream, and maintains access to fuel beyond the current moment. It is one way the system extends stability across time.

Insulin also helps coordinate internal release. When external fuel is entering the system, the liver does not need to release glucose in the same way it might during fasting or absence of input. Insulin signaling helps communicate that incoming fuel is available, allowing internal release to be reduced or adjusted. This prevents the system from adding too much glucose while also processing incoming supply.

The coordination between incoming fuel and liver glucose release is essential. If food input appears while internal release continues strongly, circulating availability can become higher or more prolonged than the immediate input alone would suggest. If internal release decreases appropriately, incoming fuel can be handled with less overlap. Insulin helps coordinate that transition.

This does not make insulin a single switch. Internal release is influenced by multiple signals, including counter-regulatory signals that preserve availability when needed. Insulin participates in the balance by supporting storage and uptake while helping reduce the need for internal supply. The pattern depends on how these signals interact.

Insulin also shapes metabolic direction. Metabolic direction refers to the system's current orientation toward receiving, distributing, storing, preserving, or releasing fuel. When incoming energy is present, insulin helps shift the system toward handling that energy. This shift includes uptake into tissues, storage for later, and reduced reliance on internal release.

Direction is broader than momentary glucose lowering. A single reading may show that blood sugar is declining, but the underlying system may be shifting from a supply-preservation state into a fuel-handling state. Insulin helps organize that shift. It informs tissues that fuel has arrived and that the system can adjust away from internal provision toward integration of incoming energy.

Timing is central to this coordination. Insulin signaling must align with glucose availability, tissue demand, and internal release. A well-timed signal supports smoother regulation because it appears when tissues need to respond and when incoming fuel must be distributed. The system can then move glucose toward use or storage while adjusting internal supply.

When timing is mismatched, regulation may require more effort. A delayed signal can allow glucose to remain elevated longer before clearance becomes effective. A prolonged signal can keep the system oriented toward uptake or storage beyond the immediate need. A signal that is poorly interpreted by tissues may require additional adjustment cycles before blood sugar returns toward the working range.

These timing issues should not be interpreted as moral failures or isolated defects. They are system coordination problems. Blood sugar stability depends on timing across loops: when glucose appears, when insulin signaling rises, how tissues respond, when liver release changes, and how counter-regulatory signals adjust. Insulin is part of that timing structure.

Insulin also functions as a translation signal between availability and action. Glucose appearing in circulation does not automatically determine where it should go, how quickly it should move, or whether it should be used immediately or stored for later. Those decisions are not conscious decisions, but they are regulatory distinctions the system must make. Insulin helps translate the presence of available fuel into a coordinated response across tissues.

This translation role is important because the same glucose availability can require different handling in different contexts. Incoming fuel after a period of higher demand may be directed more readily toward tissues that can use or store it. Incoming fuel during a state of lower demand may require a different balance between uptake, storage, and continued availability. Insulin helps organize that response, but the final pattern depends on how the whole system interprets the signal.

Tissue response determines how insulin's signal is expressed. The same signal may produce different outcomes depending on demand and capacity. A system with greater tissue demand may clear glucose more readily. A system under stress, sleep disruption, or low recovery may interpret the signal differently. Prior conditions shape responsiveness before insulin arrives.

This explains why insulin alone cannot account for blood sugar behavior. A signal is only one side of regulation. The receiving tissue, the current baseline tendency, internal release, and system constraints all contribute to the visible pattern. Insulin may be necessary for coordination, but it is not sufficient as a full explanation.

Counter-regulatory signaling provides the other side of the control environment. While insulin generally supports uptake, storage, and reduced release, counter-regulatory signals support glucose availability when needed. They help preserve supply during fasting, stress, and demand states. Blood sugar stability depends on coordination between these opposing but complementary signals.

This pairing is not a conflict between good and bad signals. It is a control system. One set of signals helps move glucose out of circulation when fuel is available. Another helps maintain or raise availability when supply is needed. Stability emerges from their coordination, not from the dominance of one signal over the other.

Insulin can be misread when it is isolated from this paired structure. Fear-based interpretations often treat insulin as something to suppress rather than as a necessary signal for handling fuel. This view turns a regulatory messenger into a problem. It also obscures the fact that glucose stability depends on both storage and release, both uptake and availability.

A more accurate interpretation places insulin within the system's communication layer. Insulin informs tissues that glucose availability has changed. It helps coordinate movement into cells, supports storage, and contributes to reduced internal release when external supply is present. Its role is not moral, and it is not ideological. It is regulatory.

The Insulin Regulation Mechanism therefore connects input, output, and internal release. When food introduces fuel, insulin helps organize handling. When tissues need to take up glucose, insulin helps coordinate clearance. When the liver is releasing glucose, insulin helps signal whether that release should continue or adjust. The signal links these layers into a more coherent response.

Blood sugar stability depends on insulin signaling that is proportionate, timely, and interpreted within context. Proportionate signaling helps match the size and duration of the response to the availability of glucose. Timely signaling helps align uptake and storage with appearance. Contextual interpretation ensures that the same signal is understood in relation to demand, recovery, stress load, and baseline state.

When insulin coordination is smooth, the system can shift from receiving fuel to distributing and storing it without excessive regulatory strain. When coordination is delayed, prolonged, or constrained, blood sugar may remain elevated longer, decline unevenly, or require more adjustment to return toward range. The difference lies in the quality of coordination across the system.

Insulin is therefore central but not solitary. It supports stability by helping the system handle glucose availability, but it must operate alongside tissue demand, internal release, counter-regulation, recovery capacity, and constraint. It is one side of a broader control system, and its meaning becomes complete only when understood alongside the signals that preserve or raise glucose availability when needed.

The Counter-Regulation Mechanism

Blood sugar regulation requires signals that preserve availability, not only signals that lower circulating glucose. If regulation were only a process of moving glucose out of circulation, the system would be incomplete. Glucose must be cleared when availability exceeds immediate need, but it must also remain accessible when food is absent, delayed, or insufficient for current demand. Stability depends on both removal and preservation.

This distinction is often missed because blood sugar stability is commonly misunderstood as a downward problem. In that narrow frame, a rise is treated as the main event, and lowering becomes the central goal. Any signal that increases glucose availability can then appear disruptive. But blood sugar cannot be regulated only by lowering. A system that only clears glucose would eventually compromise availability.

This is the missing half of many blood sugar interpretations. The visible concern is often excess, because excess is easier to notice on a chart or in a measured value. But the system is not designed only to avoid excess. It is also designed to avoid insufficient availability. A regulated variable must be defended from both sides. Too much movement upward can create instability, but too much downward movement can also create instability if tissues no longer have reliable access to fuel.

Counter-regulation becomes understandable when blood sugar is viewed through this two-sided requirement. The system must be able to remove glucose when availability exceeds immediate need, but it must also be able to preserve or restore glucose when availability is threatened. Stability is not the absence of glucose-raising signals. It is the coordination of those signals with the conditions that call for them.

The Counter-Regulation Mechanism explains the availability-preserving side of blood sugar control. Counter-regulation refers to signals that help maintain or raise glucose availability when the system needs access to fuel. These signals support internal release, protect against excessive decline, and help maintain a functional working range during fasting, stress, activity, sleep-wake transitions, and other demand states.

Counter-regulation is not outside the system. It is not a contradiction of regulation. It is regulation moving in the other direction. Just as insulin signaling helps coordinate uptake, storage, and reduced internal release when fuel is available, counter-regulatory signaling helps preserve supply when availability needs support. These are paired control layers, not opposing moral categories.

The paired nature of these signals is essential. Insulin generally helps the system move glucose into tissues and storage when incoming fuel is present. Counter-regulatory signals help the system maintain access to glucose when external input is absent or demand increases. One side supports clearance and storage. The other supports availability and release. Stability requires their coordination.

This pairing prevents blood sugar regulation from becoming one-directional. The system cannot simply lower glucose whenever it appears. It must interpret whether glucose should be removed, preserved, released, or made more available. The answer depends on context: current demand, fasting state, stress load, sleep and recovery, tissue uptake, baseline tendency, and prior conditions.

Glucose availability must be protected because tissues continue functioning between meals, overnight, during fasting intervals, and under changing demand. Cellular work does not pause when food is absent.

Organs continue their work, tissues continue using fuel, and the system continues maintaining baseline function. If glucose were only cleared and never supported internally, availability could fall below the range needed for continuity.

Counter-regulation helps prevent that by supporting fuel access when external input is limited. It helps maintain circulating glucose while tissues continue removing it. This does not mean glucose must always rise. It means the system has mechanisms to defend availability when removal continues and incoming fuel is not present.

This defense against excessive decline is as important as clearance after excess. If tissue uptake continued without adequate replacement, the system would gradually lose circulating availability. Counter-regulatory signaling helps prevent that by creating a supply response when removal, demand, or absence of input would otherwise lower availability too far. In this sense, the glucose-raising side of regulation protects continuity.

That protection can appear quiet when it is well matched. Blood sugar may remain steady across a fasting interval not because the system is inactive, but because release and uptake are being balanced. The measured value may look uneventful, while underneath it, one layer is removing glucose and another is preserving it. Counter-regulation helps make that quiet stability possible.

The liver is central to this availability-preserving role. Counter-regulatory signals can support liver glucose release when the system needs internal supply. During low-input states, internal release helps maintain circulation even though food is not entering. This allows blood sugar to remain regulated across gaps in intake rather than becoming entirely dependent on recent meals.

Internal release and tissue uptake operate at the same time. Tissues may continue drawing glucose from circulation while the liver contributes glucose back into circulation. Blood sugar reflects the relationship between these two movements. A stable level during fasting may therefore represent active balance, not inactivity.

Fasting makes counter-regulation more visible because external input is absent. In that state, the system relies more heavily on internal release and availability-preserving signals. Counter-regulation helps maintain the working range while tissues continue to use glucose. The absence of food does not mean the absence of regulation; it shifts the source of regulation toward internal supply.

This is why fasting blood sugar cannot be interpreted only as leftover input. It may reflect ongoing release, tissue uptake, signal timing, and demand. The system is maintaining availability in the absence of incoming fuel. Counter-regulation helps explain how blood sugar can remain stable, or sometimes rise, when no food has been consumed.

Stress makes the mechanism visible in another way. Stress can signal demand or threat, and the system may respond by preserving or increasing glucose availability. This response prepares fuel access for a perceived need. A rise in blood sugar under stress can therefore reflect demand-oriented regulation rather than food input.

This does not make stress-related glucose movement a moral failure or a sign that regulation has stopped. It means the system is interpreting conditions and adjusting availability. The same signaling that helps preserve function under demand can also change the visible glucose pattern. Blood sugar rises without food when internal supply is mobilized.

The morning transition also illustrates counter-regulation. Overnight, the system maintains glucose availability while external input is absent. As waking approaches, demand changes. The body moves from sleep regulation toward alertness, movement, and engagement. Availability-preserving signals may contribute to internal release as the system prepares for the shift.

Morning glucose patterns can therefore reflect transition, not only prior food. The system is moving between regulatory states. Counter-regulatory signaling may help increase availability for waking demand, while insulin signaling and tissue uptake continue shaping how glucose is handled. The visible pattern reflects coordination across this transition.

Counter-regulation does not operate separately from output. Tissues continue removing glucose even when availability-preserving signals are active. The system must balance release with uptake. If tissue demand is high, more glucose may be removed. If internal release increases, availability may be supported. Blood sugar reflects the ongoing relationship between these processes.

This relationship makes counter-regulation a balancing mechanism rather than simply a glucose-raising mechanism. Its purpose is not to raise glucose without limit. Its role is to preserve availability relative to demand. The same signal that supports stability in one context could contribute to variability in another if it becomes prolonged or mismatched.

Coordination with insulin is therefore necessary. If insulin signaling dominates when availability needs preservation, glucose may decline more than the system can comfortably support. If counter-regulatory signaling remains strong when uptake and storage should become more prominent, glucose may stay elevated longer. Stability depends on timing and proportion rather than on either side acting alone.

Timing determines whether a signal supports the current need. Counter-regulation during fasting or demand can preserve availability. The same availability-preserving signal after incoming fuel has arrived may need to taper so uptake and storage can proceed. The system must shift between preserving and clearing as conditions change.

Proportion matters as well. A small increase in internal release may support availability without creating excessive movement. A stronger or prolonged signal may produce a larger rise or longer elevation. This does not make the signal harmful by nature. It means the stability value of the signal depends on how well it matches demand.

Constraints can alter this matching. Sleep disruption, chronic stress load, low recovery capacity, illness-like strain, or repeated volatility can affect how counter-regulatory signals appear and resolve. The system may still be regulating, but it may require more effort to balance release and uptake. The visible pattern may become more variable because the control layers are operating under constraint.

Counter-regulation changes interpretation. A rise in blood sugar does not always mean food caused it. It may reflect the system preserving availability. A stable fasting level does not mean nothing is happening. It may reflect a dynamic balance between liver glucose release and tissue uptake. A morning rise does not require a food explanation to be meaningful within regulation.

This interpretation reduces the tendency to treat glucose-raising signals as failures. The system must be able to raise or preserve glucose when needed. Stability is not permanent suppression of movement. It is the ability to maintain a functional range across changing conditions, including conditions where availability must be defended.

The Counter-Regulation Mechanism also clarifies why blood sugar can become more variable when demand and signaling are mismatched. If availability is preserved when demand is present, the response may support continuity. If availability continues after demand has passed, or if release exceeds what tissues are removing, glucose may remain elevated longer. The issue is not that counter-regulation exists, but whether it is coordinated.

This distinction keeps the mechanism from being misread as either good or bad. A glucose-raising signal can support stability when availability is genuinely needed, and the same kind of signal can contribute to volatility when it persists beyond the need or appears out of proportion to the demand. The meaning of the signal depends on timing, duration, and context.

That is why counter-regulation cannot be judged by direction alone. A rise may be appropriate if the system is defending availability, preparing for demand, or compensating for continued tissue uptake. A prolonged rise may indicate that the release side of regulation is not tapering cleanly relative to uptake and storage. The difference is not the existence of glucose-raising signaling; it is whether the signal remains integrated with the rest of the control system.

Insulin and counter-regulatory signaling together form a control system. One side helps handle incoming fuel through uptake, storage, and reduced release. The other helps preserve availability through internal release and protection from excessive decline. Neither side explains blood sugar stability alone.

Blood sugar is a regulated variable because both directions are available to the system. It can move glucose out of circulation when fuel is abundant, and it can add or preserve glucose when supply is needed. The working range is maintained through these adjustments, not through one signal dominating the other.

Stability across time depends on the balance between glucose-lowering and glucose-raising forces. Clearance without preservation would threaten availability. Preservation without clearance would create prolonged elevation. The system requires both sides, coordinated by timing, proportion, demand, and context, so that blood sugar can remain available without becoming uncontrolled.

The Balance Mechanism

Blood sugar stability depends on opposing forces that are not enemies. One side helps move glucose out of circulation when availability is sufficient. The other helps preserve or raise glucose availability when supply is needed. These forces move in different directions, but their purpose is shared. They keep blood sugar within a functional range across changing conditions.

The Balance Mechanism explains how glucose-lowering and glucose-raising forces coordinate across time. Insulin-supported uptake, storage, and reduced internal release help handle glucose when fuel is available. Counter-regulatory signals help preserve availability through internal release and protection against excessive decline. Tissue demand, liver output, timing, proportion, and constraint determine how these forces interact.

Balance is often misunderstood because it is imagined as stillness or equality. In blood sugar regulation, balance does not mean both sides apply equal pressure at every moment. The system may lean toward clearance after incoming fuel, toward preservation during fasting, or toward release during stress or demand. Stability comes from appropriate shifting, not constant sameness.

A stable system is not one that refuses movement. It is one that can move in the correct direction, at the correct scale, for the correct duration, and then adjust again as conditions change. Blood sugar may rise, decline, plateau, or transition while remaining regulated. The question is not whether movement occurs, but whether movement remains coordinated around the working range.

Glucose-lowering forces contribute to balance by preventing prolonged excess when glucose availability rises. When fuel enters circulation, insulin signaling helps coordinate tissue uptake and storage. It also helps reduce the need for liver glucose release when incoming fuel is available. These actions help move glucose away from unmanaged circulation and toward use or reserve.

This does not make lowering inherently superior. Lowering is useful when it matches availability and demand. If glucose has appeared and tissues can receive it, clearance supports stability. But if availability needs to be preserved, excessive lowering would be poorly matched to the system's needs. Direction only has meaning in context.

Glucose-raising forces contribute to balance from the opposite direction. Counter-regulatory signaling helps preserve or increase glucose availability when the system requires access to fuel. During fasting, stress, morning transition, activity demand, or low input, these signals support internal release and help protect against excessive decline.

This does not make raising inherently disruptive. Raising is useful when availability must be defended. A rise can be part of regulation when it supplies the system during demand or absence of input. The stability question is not whether glucose rises, but whether the rise is proportionate, timely, and recoverable.

Insulin and counter-regulatory signaling are paired control layers. They can oppose each other directionally while still belonging to the same system. One supports uptake, storage, and reduced release. The other supports availability, release, and protection from decline. Opposition is not the same as conflict. A system often requires opposing movements to maintain range.

The distinction matters because blood sugar regulation cannot be understood by favoring one direction permanently. If insulin-supported clearance dominated without regard to need, availability could fall too far. If counter-regulatory preservation dominated without regard to incoming fuel and tissue uptake, glucose could remain elevated too long. Balance requires movement between directions.

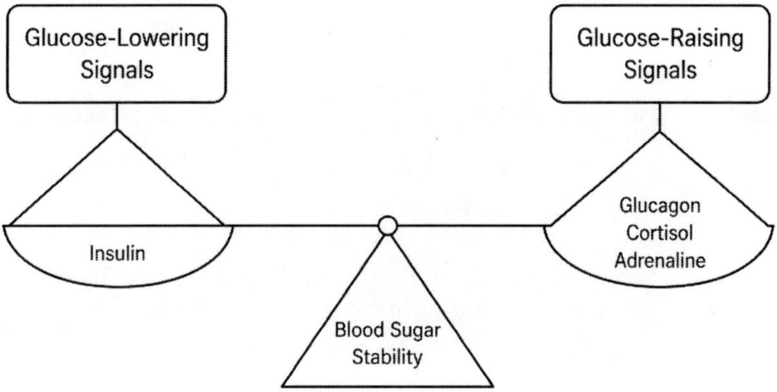

[Figure 5: Insulin and Counter-Regulation Balance]

The balance scale is useful only if it is not interpreted too literally. Blood sugar stability does not require both sides to weigh the same at every moment. The image represents relationship, not permanent equality. One side may become more active after food input, while the other may become more active during fasting, stress, or demand. The fulcrum is stability because stability depends on the system's ability to shift weight without losing coordination.

In this sense, balance is closer to controlled adjustment than fixed symmetry. The system is constantly redistributing emphasis between uptake and release, storage and availability, lowering and preserving. The point is not to freeze the scale in the middle. The point is to keep the movement organized enough that blood sugar remains within a functional range.

The relationship between tissue uptake and liver release is central to this balance. Tissues remove glucose from circulation for use, storage, and ongoing function. The liver can add glucose to circulation when availability needs support. Blood sugar at any moment reflects the relationship between these two movements, not one movement alone.

A stable level can therefore represent active motion in both directions. Tissues may be taking up glucose while the liver releases enough to maintain availability. The visible number may appear steady, but underneath it, removal and supply are both operating. Stability is not inactivity. It is coordinated exchange.

After food input, the balance may shift toward tissue uptake and storage. The system has incoming fuel to handle, and glucose-lowering forces may become more prominent. During fasting or demand, the balance may shift toward internal release. The system has less external input available, so glucose-raising forces may preserve supply. Neither state is morally better. Each reflects a different regulatory need.

Timing determines whether a signal supports stability or creates mismatch. Glucose-lowering signals need to rise in relation to glucose appearance, tissue readiness, and storage demand. They also need to resolve as the need for clearance changes. If they arrive too late, glucose may remain elevated longer. If they continue too long, availability may be pulled lower than needed.

Glucose-raising signals also depend on timing. During fasting, morning transition, stress, or demand, they may help preserve availability. Once incoming fuel is present or demand has changed, those signals may need to taper. If they remain strong after the need has passed, the system may continue adding glucose when clearance would be more appropriate.

Proportion adds another layer. A response can be directionally correct but too small, too large, too short, or too prolonged. Too little lowering may allow glucose to remain elevated after availability rises. Too much lowering may create pressure in the opposite direction. Too little raising may fail to preserve availability during absence of input. Too much raising may prolong elevation beyond current demand.

Proportion is not about perfect symmetry. It is about fit. The size and duration of a response should match the system state. A small rise in availability may require a modest clearance response. A larger or faster appearance may require more coordinated uptake and storage. A brief demand state may require temporary preservation. A prolonged demand state may require sustained internal support.

This is why balance differs from flatness. A flat line can appear stable, but biological stability is not defined by visual stillness. A regulated system must be able to shift. It must make glucose available, remove glucose, store fuel, reduce release, increase release, and return toward range as conditions change.

Balance means those shifts remain coherent. Movement should be recoverable. A rise should not automatically become prolonged. A decline should not become excessive. A preservation response should not remain stronger than the demand that required it. A clearance response should not continue beyond the context that made it useful.

Constraints can affect every part of this process. Stress load, sleep disruption, low recovery capacity, reduced tissue demand, aging, repeated volatility, and prior conditions can change how signals are produced, interpreted, and resolved. Under constraint, the same signal may become slower, stronger, weaker, prolonged, or less precisely matched to need.

Constraint does not remove regulation. It changes the cost and quality of regulation. The system may still lower glucose, raise glucose, preserve availability, and support uptake, but it may require more effort to do so. Responses may become less flexible. Transitions may become less smooth. The working range may become harder to maintain.

This added effort matters because a system can still appear regulated while becoming less efficient at regulation. Blood sugar may return toward range, but only after a longer delay, a stronger signal, or a larger counter-response. The visible result may look like a normal correction if viewed once, but repeated patterns can reveal that balance is being maintained with less margin.

A lower-margin system is not unregulated. It is more sensitive to disruption. Smaller changes in input, demand, sleep, stress, or timing may produce larger visible movement because the opposing sides of regulation no longer adjust as smoothly. Balance is still present, but it is less forgiving. The same forces remain available, but their coordination has become more costly.

Imbalance can appear in several forms. Glucose may remain elevated longer because clearance is delayed, internal release continues, or tissue uptake is constrained. Glucose may decline more sharply because clearance exceeds current availability. Recovery may take longer because signals do not resolve cleanly. Variability may widen because the system is repeatedly shifting between opposing responses.

Overcorrection is one expression of imbalance. A response intended to restore range can move too far in the opposite direction, requiring another adjustment. This can create oscillation, where the system alternates between correction and counter-correction rather than resolving smoothly. The problem is not that either signal exists. The problem is that timing and proportion have become mismatched.

Prolonged elevation reflects another pattern. If glucose-raising forces remain active while input is present, or if tissue uptake is constrained while liver output continues, blood sugar may stay above the working range longer than expected. This pattern reflects the relationship between supply and removal, not a single cause.

Excessive decline reflects the opposite mismatch. If glucose-lowering forces exceed the current need or continue beyond the availability they were meant to handle, the system may need counter-regulatory support to preserve function. The resulting pattern may look unstable, but it is still built from regulatory signals attempting to maintain range.

The Balance Mechanism changes interpretation by shifting attention away from one-direction explanations. Blood sugar is not stable because lowering wins. It is not stable because raising is suppressed. It is stable when lowering and raising forces remain coordinated with demand, availability, tissue response, and internal release.

This framework also prevents moral interpretation. A rise is not automatically failure. A decline is not automatically success. A glucose-raising signal is not bad, and a glucose-lowering signal is not good in isolation. Each signal has a role only in relation to timing, proportion, and context.

Blood sugar stability requires both sides of regulation to remain available. The system needs insulin-supported uptake and storage when glucose appears. It needs counter-regulatory preservation and release when availability must be protected. It needs tissue uptake to remove glucose and liver output to supply it. Stability depends on the capacity to shift between these roles.

Balance across time is therefore dynamic control, not a static midpoint. The system moves between clearance and preservation, storage and release, uptake and supply. When these movements are matched to context, blood sugar remains more coherent. When one side responds too strongly, too late, or too long, balance can turn into overcorrection.

The Overcorrection Mechanism

A correction can be necessary and still overshoot. Blood sugar regulation depends on responses that move glucose back toward a working range when availability rises, falls, or drifts. The system must correct change. Without correction, glucose would accumulate when availability is high, fall too far when supply is low, or remain poorly matched to demand. Correction is not the problem. The problem begins when a correction moves beyond what the current situation requires.

The Overcorrection Mechanism explains how a regulatory response can become excessive relative to need. A response may be directionally appropriate but too strong, too late, too prolonged, or poorly matched to the system state. Glucose-lowering forces may continue after the original rise has already changed. Glucose-raising forces may respond strongly after a decline. The system is still regulating, but the response is no longer proportionate to the condition it is trying to resolve.

This distinction matters because overcorrection is often misunderstood through experience rather than mechanism. A sharp decline may be described as a crash. A sudden shift in appetite, urgency, fatigue, irritability, or craving may be interpreted as weakness, poor discipline, or a behavioral problem. But these patterns can also reflect feedback dynamics. They can emerge when the system attempts to restore range and overshoots, creating a new need for correction in the opposite direction.

Correction is built into regulation. When glucose appears in circulation, insulin-supported uptake and storage help move it toward tissues and reserve. When glucose availability is threatened, counter-regulatory signals help preserve or raise supply. These responses are necessary because blood sugar is a regulated variable, not a passive number. The system must be able to move in both directions.

Overcorrection occurs when that movement exceeds the need. A response designed to bring glucose down may continue after sufficient clearance has already occurred. A response designed to preserve availability may remain active after the demand has changed. A signal may arrive later than ideal, forcing a stronger adjustment than would have been required earlier. The mismatch is not the presence of response, but the fit of response.

Timing is one path into overshoot. If a glucose-lowering response arrives late, blood sugar may rise farther before clearance becomes effective. The system may then respond more forcefully to a larger movement. By the time uptake and storage accelerate, the original condition may already be changing. The response can carry momentum past the intended return toward range.

Proportion is another path. A response may be correctly directed but too large in scale or duration. Glucose-lowering forces may exceed the current amount of circulating availability. Counter-regulatory signals may raise availability more than the demand requires. The system is attempting to restore balance, but the magnitude of the response becomes mismatched to the actual state.

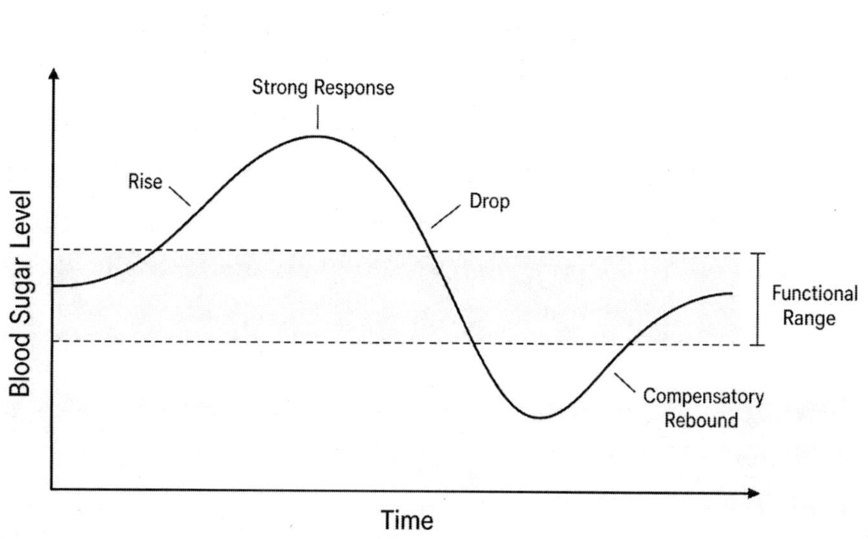

[Figure 6: Overcorrection Pattern]

The pattern is important because it shows that instability can emerge from correction itself. The initial rise is not the entire story. The strong response that follows may be intended to restore range, but if it continues with too much force or for too long, the line can move below the functional range instead of settling within it. The compensatory rebound then becomes another attempt to restore availability after the previous response overshot.

This makes overcorrection different from a simple rise-and-fall pattern. In a smooth correction, movement returns toward range and resolves. In an overcorrection pattern, the response creates a new disturbance that the system must address. The system is not inactive or broken; it is caught in a sequence where each adjustment creates the need for another adjustment.

A glucose-lowering overshoot can contribute to the pattern commonly experienced as a crash. If insulin-supported uptake, storage, and reduced internal release combine in a way that removes glucose faster or longer than the system needs, circulating availability may decline sharply. The visible pattern may be a drop, but the underlying mechanism is a correction that has moved too far.

A crash should not be interpreted as proof that regulation has disappeared. It is often evidence that regulation is active but poorly matched in timing or proportion. The system responded to glucose availability, but the response did not settle smoothly into the working range. Instead, it moved through the range and created pressure in the opposite direction.

That pressure can produce urgency because the system is defending availability. A sharper decline can be interpreted internally as a need for fuel access. The resulting urgency is not irrationality or character failure. It reflects the body's prioritization of restoring usable supply when availability appears threatened or insufficient for current demand.

Urgency may take different forms. It may appear as hunger, craving, fatigue, restlessness, or a strong drive toward intake. These experiences can be moralized when viewed only through behavior. Through the Overcorrection Mechanism, they become more understandable as signals emerging from a system trying to correct a perceived or actual shortage.

Compensatory responses can follow the same logic. When blood sugar declines too sharply or availability feels unstable, the system may generate stronger signals to restore access to fuel. These responses are not separate from regulation. They are part of the attempt to protect function after a prior correction has exceeded the need.

Counter-regulatory signaling often participates after a glucose-lowering overshoot. If availability falls too far or too quickly, glucose-raising signals may increase internal release to defend the working range. The liver may release glucose, and the system may shift toward preservation rather than clearance. This rebound is not random chaos. It is a counter-correction.

The rebound pattern becomes important because it shows how overcorrection can create additional movement rather than resolution. A rise may be followed by a strong lowering response. The decline may then trigger glucose-raising support. The result is not smooth recovery but alternating correction and counter-correction. Blood sugar becomes more variable because the system keeps responding to its own overshoot.

This oscillation is different from ordinary movement. Blood sugar movement is normal. A rise after input, a decline after uptake, a maintained level during fasting, or an increase during demand can all be part of regulation. Overcorrection refers to movement that exceeds what the working range and current demand require. It is not the existence of change but the loss of proportion within change.

The working range gives movement its meaning. A decline is not automatically unstable. A rebound is not automatically failure. Each pattern must be understood relative to timing, demand, baseline tendency, tissue uptake, internal release, and recovery. Overcorrection appears when the system moves past the intended return and creates a new regulatory problem.

Constraints can increase the likelihood of overshoot by reducing regulatory margin. When recovery capacity is low, stress load is high, sleep is disrupted, or prior volatility has accumulated, the system may have less room for precise adjustment. Signals may become stronger, slower, or more prolonged because the system is working under pressure.

A fasting state can also alter the margin around correction. When external input is absent, internal release and counter-regulatory signaling help preserve availability. If glucose-lowering forces become prominent in that context, the system may respond defensively. If glucose-raising signals become strong, availability may rebound. The same mechanisms are present, but the starting state changes how they behave.

Low tissue demand can affect the pattern from another direction. If tissues are not removing glucose readily, blood sugar may remain elevated longer, prompting stronger or prolonged lowering signals. If clearance eventually becomes more active than needed, the system may move into decline. Output capacity and timing therefore shape whether correction resolves smoothly or overshoots.

Stress load can intensify counter-correction. When the system is already oriented toward availability, a decline may be met with stronger glucose-raising signals. The body may prioritize access to fuel under perceived demand. This can produce rebound patterns that reflect stress-state regulation rather than a simple response to food.

Sleep and recovery influence signal interpretation as well. Disrupted recovery can alter baseline tendency, tissue responsiveness, and the timing of glucose-raising or glucose-lowering signals. Under these conditions, the system may still correct, but corrections may be less precise. More regulatory effort may be required to achieve the same return toward range.

Overcorrection changes interpretation by separating experience from blame. A crash does not need to be framed as weakness. Urgency does not need to be framed as lack of discipline. Compensatory behavior does not need to be reduced to failure. These patterns can arise from feedback loops trying to restore availability after a mismatch in timing or proportion.

This does not mean every sensation or response can be explained by blood sugar alone. The point is narrower and more structural: when glucose regulation overshoots, the system may produce signals and behaviors that reflect availability defense. The mechanism provides a way to understand these patterns without turning them into moral judgments.

The Overcorrection Mechanism also clarifies why stronger responses are not always more stable. A powerful glucose-lowering response may appear effective if the only goal is to reduce a rise quickly. But if that response pushes availability too far downward, it can create the need for a counter-response. Stability depends on resolution, not force.

The same applies to glucose-raising forces. A strong counter-regulatory response may preserve availability after a sharp decline, but if it continues beyond the demand, it can prolong elevation or widen variability. The value of a signal depends on fit. Direction alone does not determine whether a response supports stability.

Stable regulation requires correction without excessive carryover. Glucose-lowering forces need to move availability toward use, storage, and range without overshooting into perceived shortage. Glucose-raising forces need to preserve availability without continuing beyond the need. Both sides must appear, scale, and resolve in relation to context.

When overcorrection repeats, the system can become more effortful to regulate. Each overshoot creates another condition requiring response. A rise prompts lowering, lowering produces decline, decline prompts raising, and raising may prolong elevation. The system remains active, but its activity becomes less efficient and more variable.

This repeated effort matters because regulation has a cost. Each correction requires signal production, tissue response, release adjustment, and recovery toward range. When corrections resolve smoothly, the system returns toward ordinary regulation with less carryover. When corrections repeatedly overshoot, the system spends more time managing the consequences of prior responses. The control system remains active, but more of its activity is spent resolving instability rather than maintaining quiet continuity.

Repeated overcorrection can also alter the baseline environment. If the system frequently has to defend availability or recover from prolonged movement, it may operate with higher regulatory effort. The working range may become less settled, and the margin for smooth adjustment may narrow. Over time, unresolved overshoot can contribute to a pattern in which stability requires more correction, more counter-correction, and more effort to maintain.

The Baseline Elevation Mechanism

Blood sugar can change not only by rising and falling in the moment, but by drifting upward in its ordinary return point over time. A rise after input, a decline after clearance, or a temporary increase during stress can all occur within normal regulation. Baseline elevation is different. It describes a shift in the level the system tends to return toward after those movements resolve.

The Baseline Elevation Mechanism explains this gradual upward drift. It is not a single reading, a single spike, or one visible event. It is a pattern across time in which the resting tendency moves higher and regulation requires more effort to maintain the working range. Blood sugar may still rise and fall, but the starting point and return point become less settled than before.

This distinction matters because baseline elevation is easily misunderstood. A higher ordinary pattern may be interpreted as sudden failure, a food-only issue, or a personal discipline problem. That interpretation compresses a time-based regulatory pattern into a single cause. Baseline elevation is better understood as the result of interacting forces: internal release, tissue uptake, insulin signaling, counter-regulatory signaling, stress load, sleep and recovery, repeated correction, and constraint.

Fluctuation is movement around a range. Baseline is the underlying tendency around which that movement occurs. A system can fluctuate without drifting. Blood sugar can rise, decline, and return while the ordinary baseline remains stable. In that case, variation is contained within a working range that remains relatively consistent across time.

Baseline elevation begins when the return point itself shifts upward. The system still corrects. It still clears glucose. It still releases glucose internally. It still uses signals to preserve availability and prevent excessive decline. But the range around which these processes organize becomes higher, often with greater regulatory effort beneath the surface.

A spike is acute movement. Drift is slow movement in the underlying pattern. A spike may be noticeable because it rises quickly and resolves visibly. Drift can be less obvious because it develops gradually. No single moment may appear dramatic, yet the ordinary baseline may be moving upward across repeated cycles.

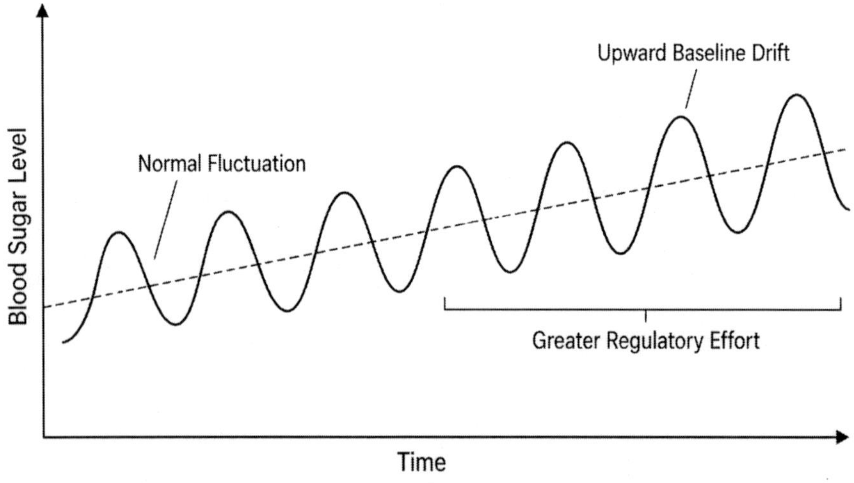

[Figure 7: Baseline Elevation]

The figure is useful because it separates visible fluctuation from underlying drift. The repeated rises and declines show ordinary movement, but the gradually rising baseline shows that the system is returning to a different starting point over time. The important feature is not one peak or one low point. It is the upward movement of the line that the fluctuations are organized around.

This is why baseline elevation can be missed when attention stays on isolated readings. One day may look similar to another. One rise may resolve. One decline may appear reassuring. But if the return point gradually moves upward, the system's ordinary operating state has changed even though daily movement continues to look familiar.

The difference between a spike and drift changes interpretation. A spike asks what produced a temporary movement. Drift asks why the system's ordinary starting point has changed. The first concerns a moment. The second concerns the operating state of regulation across time.

Baseline elevation does not mean regulation has disappeared. It often means regulation is still active but more effortful. The system may continue clearing glucose into tissues, reducing internal release when appropriate, preserving availability when needed, and correcting movement back toward range. The issue is that this regulation may now occur from a higher baseline and with a narrower margin for clean adjustment.

Regulatory effort refers to how much signal activity, tissue response, internal release adjustment, and recovery are required to maintain the working range. A system with more margin may correct ordinary movement with less visible disturbance. A system requiring more effort may still correct, but the correction takes more signal intensity, more time, or more counter-adjustment.

This matters because effort can rise before regulation appears obviously unstable. Blood sugar may still move back toward range, but the return may be slower, more conditional, or more dependent on stronger opposing signals. The system continues to regulate, but the cost of maintaining that regulation has increased.

Internal release can contribute to that upward pull. The liver releases glucose to preserve availability during fasting states, morning transitions, stress, demand, and low-input periods. This internal supply is essential to regulation. But when release remains more active than the situation requires, or when it resolves less cleanly, the baseline tendency can be pulled higher.

This does not make internal release a defect. It is a protective layer of regulation. The problem is not release itself but persistence, timing, and proportion. Availability support that is useful during absence of input can contribute to baseline elevation if it becomes prolonged, mismatched, or repeatedly activated under constraint.

Tissue uptake forms the other side of the pattern. If tissues are slower to receive glucose, less responsive to signals, or operating under reduced demand, glucose can remain in circulation longer. Output still exists, but it may be constrained. The system may require more time, stronger signaling, or repeated adjustment to move glucose toward use or storage.

Constrained uptake can gradually affect the ordinary return point. If glucose remains elevated longer after repeated inputs or internal release episodes, the system spends more time operating above its prior baseline. Over time, that repeated exposure can make the higher state feel more ordinary within the regulatory pattern. The baseline does not jump; it drifts.

Repeated overcorrection can intensify the same effect. When a strong correction produces a sharp decline, counter-regulatory signals may respond to preserve availability. If this rise-and-counter-rise pattern repeats, the system remains more active. It spends more time correcting, defending, rebounding, and rebalancing.

A system that repeatedly has to defend availability may become less settled. The baseline environment can shift because the body is not simply returning to a quiet state after each movement. It is carrying forward the effects of repeated correction. Regulatory effort accumulates, and the ordinary starting point may become higher or more variable.

Stress load can also influence baseline elevation. Stress signals can preserve or raise glucose availability because the system interprets demand as requiring accessible fuel. When stress-state signaling is frequent or prolonged, internal release may remain more active, and tissue response may change. Blood sugar may then reflect demand signaling even when food input is not the primary explanation.

This is one reason a higher baseline cannot always be read backward to the most recent meal. The visible number may reflect the current stress environment, the degree of internal release, and the system's readiness to preserve availability. Food may still matter, but it is not the only layer producing the pattern.

Sleep disruption and low recovery capacity affect baseline through coordination. Recovery helps signals resolve, tissues respond, and regulatory loops return toward settled function. When recovery is limited, the same glucose movement may require more regulatory effort. Timing can become less precise, and the margin for smooth correction can narrow.

Morning patterns often reveal this interaction because the system is moving from overnight regulation into waking demand. Internal release, counter-regulatory signaling, and tissue uptake are already active before food appears. If sleep and recovery are disrupted, that transition may occur from a more constrained state, contributing to a higher ordinary starting point.

Regulatory margin is the space the system has for adjustment before movement becomes prolonged, exaggerated, or difficult to resolve. As baseline elevation develops, that margin can narrow. A system starting from a higher baseline has less room for additional input, stress, internal release, or demand before glucose movement becomes larger or longer-lasting.

A narrower margin changes the effect of ordinary conditions. A meal, fasting interval, poor sleep period, stress response, or demand state may produce a more pronounced pattern because the system begins from a more effortful starting point. The same challenge can require more correction when the baseline is already elevated.

This is why baseline elevation and variability often travel together. As the ordinary return point rises, smaller changes can create wider movement. The system may have to call on stronger lowering signals, stronger counter-regulatory signals, or longer adjustment cycles. Movement becomes less contained not because regulation has vanished, but because regulation has less available margin.

Baseline elevation also changes the meaning of return. A glucose pattern may appear to resolve because it declines from a higher level, but if it returns to a higher baseline than before, the underlying state has still shifted. Resolution of a single rise does not necessarily mean the ordinary operating range remains unchanged.

This distinction is important because daily movement can hide baseline drift. A person may see repeated rises and returns and assume the system is behaving the same way each time. But the return point may be gradually changing beneath those movements. The shape of the pattern may look familiar while the level around which the pattern occurs has shifted.

In that sense, baseline elevation is not found only in the moments that look dramatic. It can appear in the quiet spaces between movements: where blood sugar settles, where the next cycle begins, and how much effort is required before the system feels returned to ordinary regulation.

The Baseline Elevation Mechanism places attention on the trend beneath daily movement. Momentary rises and falls matter, but they are not the whole story. Long-term stability depends on where the system returns after those movements and how much effort is required to return there.

A higher resting tendency should not be moralized. It is not a character statement, a discipline measure, or a score attached to behavior. It is a system pattern. It reflects the relationship between supply, removal, release, signaling, recovery, and constraint across time.

The same principle applies to fasting or morning glucose patterns. A higher pattern during absence of food may not be explained by intake alone. It may reflect liver glucose release, counter-regulatory signaling, stress load, sleep disruption, reduced tissue uptake, repeated overcorrection, or lower regulatory margin. The system is active before food arrives.

Baseline elevation therefore reframes interpretation from "what caused this number?" to "what operating state is this number expressing?" A single reading may show one point, but a baseline tendency reveals how the system is organizing regulation across repeated conditions. The important feature is not the isolated value but the direction of the pattern over time.

Blood sugar stability depends on more than the ability to correct a rise. It also depends on the stability of the return point. A system that repeatedly returns to a settled baseline has more regulatory coherence than one that returns to progressively higher or more effortful starting states.

As baseline drift and regulatory effort increase, variability can become amplified. The system has less margin for clean adjustment, and each new input, demand state, stress signal, fasting interval, or recovery disruption can produce larger movement. Baseline elevation therefore opens into a broader pattern: when the return point becomes less settled, blood sugar variation itself can become harder to contain.

The Variability Amplification Mechanism

Instability does not only change where blood sugar goes; it changes how widely, how often, and how slowly it moves. A system can become less stable not only because glucose rises higher, but because movement becomes harder to contain. Peaks may become larger, declines sharper, rebounds stronger, and recovery slower. The visible issue is not one isolated movement, but the way movement begins to expand across time.

The Variability Amplification Mechanism explains how fluctuation becomes larger, more frequent, or slower to resolve when regulatory margin narrows. Blood sugar remains regulated, but regulation becomes more effortful. The system still senses, signals, clears, releases, and corrects, yet those corrections may cover more distance, occur more often, or take longer to settle.

Variability is commonly misunderstood because blood sugar movement is often interpreted through single events. A rise may be read as a reaction to food. A drop may be read as a crash. A rebound may be read as randomness. These interpretations can capture a visible moment while missing the deeper pattern: the system's movement may be widening because regulation has less margin for clean adjustment.

Ordinary fluctuation is not the same as amplified variability. Blood sugar must move as input changes, tissues remove glucose, internal release supports availability, and demand shifts. A stable system is not flat. It can rise, decline, release, clear, and return while remaining coherent.

Movement becomes amplified when it grows wider, repeats more often, or takes longer to resolve.

The first dimension is size. Amplified variability may appear as higher peaks, deeper dips, sharper declines, stronger rebounds, or wider movement around the working range. Size matters because the system must then correct across a larger distance. A larger movement requires more coordination to return toward range without overshooting again.

The second dimension is frequency. Variability can increase when corrections and counter-corrections occur more often. A rise may trigger a strong lowering response, which may trigger availability defense, which may lead to another rebound. The problem is not one movement, but repeated movement that keeps the system in a more reactive state.

The third dimension is recovery time. A movement may not be especially high or low, but it may take longer to settle. Glucose may remain elevated longer, rebound for longer, or return toward baseline more slowly. Recovery time matters because stability depends on resolution, not only on the height of a peak or depth of a decline.

Recovery time is often the hidden dimension of variability. A movement that resolves quickly may create less carryover into the next regulatory cycle. A movement that resolves slowly can overlap with the next input, the next demand state, the next stress signal, or the next fasting interval. In that case, the system is not beginning from a clean return point. It is beginning from unfinished regulation.

This overlap is one way variability becomes amplified across time. The next event does not arrive into a settled system; it arrives into a system still resolving the previous movement. The result may be a larger response, a longer correction, or a stronger counter-response than the same event would have produced under more settled conditions.

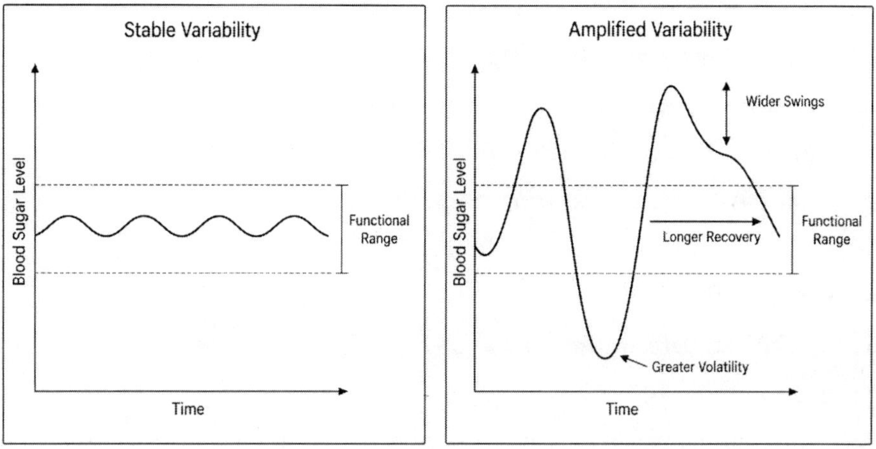

[Figure 8: Variability Amplification]

The side-by-side comparison matters because it shows that movement alone is not the problem. On the stable side, blood sugar still rises and falls, but the movement stays modest, recoverable, and contained within the functional range. On the amplified side, the same basic pattern becomes wider, slower, and more volatile. The difference is not the existence of fluctuation. The difference is the loss of containment.

This visual distinction is important because amplified variability can be misunderstood when attention focuses only on peaks. A higher peak is one sign of wider movement, but it is not the only sign. A deeper dip, a slower return, a stronger rebound, or a more frequent sequence of corrections can all indicate that the system is using more regulatory effort to manage the same basic process.

Baseline elevation can amplify variability by reducing margin. When the ordinary return point drifts upward, the system begins each new movement from a more effortful starting state. A meal, stress response, fasting interval, or demand state may produce a larger visible pattern because the system has less room to absorb additional movement.

A higher baseline also changes recovery. A decline from a peak may appear to resolve, but if it returns to a higher ordinary range, the system remains in a more effortful state. The return point matters because it determines where the next movement begins. Variability grows when each new cycle starts from a less settled baseline.

Overcorrection can amplify variability through oscillation. A response meant to restore range may move too far, creating a need for counter-correction. Glucose-lowering forces may produce a sharp decline, and glucose-raising forces may respond with rebound. The system remains active, but its activity becomes less efficient because each response creates the next disturbance.

This pattern turns regulation into repeated correction. A rise does not settle cleanly. A drop does not resolve quietly. A rebound becomes another movement requiring response. Variability expands because the system is responding not only to input, demand, or internal release, but to the consequences of its own prior corrections.

Constrained tissue uptake can widen the pattern from another direction. If tissues are slower to receive glucose relative to availability, glucose may remain in circulation longer. Clearance still occurs, but it is delayed or less effective. The visible result may be a longer elevation, slower recovery, or stronger need for later correction.

Tissue uptake depends on demand, signaling, recovery, and capacity. When output is constrained, the system may rely on stronger signaling or longer adjustment to move glucose toward use or storage. The longer glucose remains elevated, the more opportunity there is for correction to become more forceful or mistimed.

Persistent internal release can also amplify variability. Liver glucose release supports availability when food is absent or demand is present. But if internal release remains active while input is present or uptake is constrained, circulating glucose can rise higher or stay elevated longer. Internal supply then adds to the movement rather than simply maintaining continuity.

Counter-regulatory signaling is central to this process. It preserves availability when needed, but if it remains stronger than current demand requires, it can extend movement beyond the intended range. Variability increases when availability support does not taper cleanly as conditions change.

Stress load can make blood sugar more reactive by increasing demand-oriented signaling. When the system frequently interprets conditions as requiring fuel access, internal release may become more active and counter-regulatory signals may appear more often. Movement can then occur even without food input, and responses may become more frequent across the day.

This does not make stress-related movement a moral issue. It means the system is responding to perceived demand. The effect on variability depends on timing, proportion, and recovery. When demand signaling is repeated or prolonged, glucose movement can become harder to contain.

Sleep disruption and low recovery capacity affect variability by reducing precision. Recovery supports signal resolution, tissue response, and return toward baseline. When recovery is limited, glucose-lowering and glucose-raising signals may not coordinate as smoothly. Movements may become sharper, longer, or more difficult to settle.

Morning transitions can reveal this reduced precision. Overnight regulation, internal release, and waking demand overlap before food enters. If recovery is constrained, the transition may produce greater movement or a higher starting point. The pattern reflects the interaction between baseline tendency, internal release, and recovery margin.

Fasting and low-input states can also reveal variability because internal release and counter-regulation become more visible. When food is absent, tissues still remove glucose and the liver may release glucose to maintain availability. Movement during fasting does not necessarily point back to food. It may show the balance between tissue uptake, internal release, counter-regulatory signaling, and regulatory margin.

In a well-coordinated fasting state, internal release and tissue uptake may balance with relatively contained movement. Under constraint, the same state may become more variable. Availability-preserving signals may rise more strongly, tissue uptake may shift, and the return toward baseline may become slower. Fasting exposes the internal side of regulation because external input is reduced.

Variability amplification changes interpretation by shifting attention from isolated readings to pattern structure. The question is not only how high blood sugar rises or how low it falls. It is how far it moves, how often it moves, how sharply it changes, how long it takes to settle, and what baseline it returns toward afterward.

A single rise may be less meaningful than repeated rises that take longer to resolve. A single drop may be less important than a pattern of drops followed by rebounds. A stable number may be less informative than whether maintaining that number requires increasing regulatory effort. Variability is a time-based property of the system.

Pattern structure matters because two glucose movements with the same peak can have different meanings. One may rise and settle smoothly. Another may rise, stay elevated longer, decline sharply, rebound, and return to a higher baseline. The peak alone would miss the difference. The shape of the movement reveals how much regulatory effort was required and how cleanly the system recovered.

For that reason, variability amplification should be read through sequence rather than isolated moments. Size, frequency, recovery time, rebound, and return point all belong to the same pattern. Stability depends on how these features relate across time, not on whether any single number appears dramatic by itself.

The Variability Amplification Mechanism also clarifies why instability does not mean regulation has disappeared. The system may be regulating intensely. It may be producing more signals, more corrections, more internal release, and more counter-corrections. The problem is not absence of regulation, but regulation becoming wider, more frequent, and less contained.

This distinction protects the concept from moral interpretation. Wider swings, slower recovery, stronger rebounds, or sharper declines are not evidence of personal failure. They are system patterns produced by timing, proportion, demand, baseline state, recovery, and constraint. The visible movement is an output of regulation under conditions that reduce margin.

Blood sugar stability depends on contained, recoverable movement. A stable system can absorb input, support fasting, respond to stress, meet demand, and return toward its working range without excessive oscillation. Amplified variability means those movements require more effort, cover more distance, or take longer to resolve.

As variability increases, each new condition enters a less settled environment. Input arrives into a system that may already be elevated, rebounding, or defending availability. Stress signals land on a system with less margin. Fasting states may reveal more internal movement. Recovery has to resolve not one event, but a wider pattern.

This is why variability amplification becomes a bridge between daily movement and longer-term stability. The issue is not movement itself, but movement that becomes increasingly hard to contain. When the system has less margin for clean adjustment, fasting, input, internal release, counter-regulation, and recovery all interact more strongly, making the next layer of regulation more dependent on context.

The Fasting Interaction Mechanism

Fasting changes blood sugar regulation by reducing incoming fuel and making internal control more visible. When food input is present, the visible pattern is often interpreted through what has recently entered the system. When food input is absent, that explanation becomes less available. Blood sugar still moves, holds, rises, falls, or varies, but the source of those patterns becomes more clearly tied to internal release, tissue uptake, counter-regulatory signaling, insulin adjustment, demand, and recovery state.

The Fasting Interaction Mechanism explains fasting as a regulatory state. It is not an absence of regulation. It is not a pause in blood sugar control. It is a condition in which the system must maintain glucose availability without relying on incoming fuel. The balance shifts from external input handling toward internal coordination. The liver may release glucose, tissues continue removing glucose, signals adjust availability, and the working range must still be maintained.

This distinction matters because fasting is often interpreted too simply. It may be treated as if less food automatically means lower blood sugar, or as if the absence of food should produce a quiet, predictable pattern. That view misses the regulatory work that continues when input is absent. Food may be absent, but demand is not absent. Tissue use is not absent. Internal release is not absent. Signaling is not absent. The system remains active.

In a fed state, incoming fuel is more visible. Food enters, glucose availability changes, insulin signaling adjusts, tissues take up fuel, storage may increase, and internal release may shift. The visible pattern can appear tightly connected to the meal because the input is recent and identifiable. In fasting, that visible input recedes. The same regulatory system continues, but the emphasis shifts toward internal sources and internal coordination.

This shift does not make fasting inherently stabilizing or destabilizing. It changes the conditions the system must manage. Without incoming fuel, the system relies more clearly on internal release and availability-preserving signals. Whether that produces a contained pattern, a rising pattern, a declining pattern, or a more variable pattern depends on baseline tendency, tissue demand, stress load, sleep and recovery, internal release, and regulatory margin.

When food is absent, the liver becomes more visible as an internal supply layer. It can release glucose into circulation to help preserve availability. This release helps explain why blood sugar may remain stable or even rise during fasting. The absence of food does not mean the absence of glucose entering circulation. It may mean the source has shifted from external input to internal supply.

That internal supply is not a contradiction of fasting. It is part of fasting physiology. If tissues continue using glucose while no food enters, the system must have a way to prevent circulating availability from falling too far. Liver glucose release helps balance ongoing tissue uptake. It supports continuity between periods of input and prevents blood sugar from depending entirely on recent meals.

Counter-regulatory signaling becomes more visible under the same conditions. When external supply is reduced, availability-preserving signals may become more important. These signals help maintain or raise glucose availability when the system detects need, demand, or risk of decline. In fasting, their role is easier to see because food is not the obvious explanation for movement.

This does not mean counter-regulatory signaling is abnormal in fasting. It is one of the control layers that allows blood sugar to remain within a functional range. If glucose begins to fall relative to demand, or if the system anticipates need, counter-regulatory signals can support internal release. The visible result may be stability, a gradual rise, or a pattern that changes with demand and recovery.

Insulin signaling also changes in fasting, but it does not become irrelevant. Its role shifts as incoming fuel declines. With less external input to distribute, the system may reduce emphasis on storage and incoming fuel handling, while still coordinating tissue uptake and internal release. Insulin remains part of the signaling environment that helps determine whether glucose is stored, used, preserved, or released.

This is important because fasting is sometimes imagined as if one regulatory side simply turns off. The system is more precise than that. Glucose-lowering and glucose-raising signals continue to interact. Insulin signaling helps keep internal release and tissue uptake coordinated, while counter-regulatory signaling helps preserve availability. Fasting changes the balance between these signals rather than eliminating either side.

Tissue uptake continues as well. Cells do not stop requiring fuel because food is absent. Organs continue functioning, muscle tissue maintains baseline activity, and recovery processes may continue drawing on available energy. Glucose removal from circulation therefore continues during fasting. Output remains active even when input has stopped.

This ongoing output is what makes internal release necessary. If tissues remove glucose and no external fuel enters, circulating availability would decline unless internal supply compensates. Fasting blood sugar therefore reflects the balance between tissue uptake and internal release. A stable fasting pattern can represent active regulation on both sides, not inactivity.

Fasting can also reveal baseline tendency. With incoming food removed from the immediate picture, the system's ordinary return point becomes more visible. A fasting pattern may reflect internal release tendency, morning transition, stress-state signaling, recovery capacity, and the current working range. It is not simply a report on the previous meal or a measure of discipline.

Baseline elevation can shape the fasting response. If the ordinary return point has drifted upward, fasting may begin from a higher starting state. Internal release may be more active, tissue uptake may be more constrained, or regulatory effort may already be elevated. The fasting pattern then reflects the current operating state of the system, not merely the absence of food.

Fasting can also reveal variability amplification. When external input is reduced, internal control is more exposed. Movement during fasting may reflect counter-regulatory signaling, liver release, stress load, sleep disruption, tissue demand, or reduced regulatory margin. If the system has less margin for clean adjustment, fasting may make that variability more visible.

A fasting interval may therefore show stability in one context and variability in another. In one state, internal release and tissue uptake may coordinate smoothly. In another, glucose-raising signals may be stronger, tissue uptake may be slower, and return toward range may take longer. The fasting condition is the same in broad terms, but the system state is different.

The morning transition is a particularly important example. Overnight, the system maintains glucose availability without incoming food. As waking approaches, demand begins to change. The body shifts from sleep regulation toward alertness, movement, and engagement. Internal release and counter-regulatory signaling may support this transition by increasing availability before food appears.

Morning glucose patterns therefore cannot be reduced to the previous meal alone. They may reflect overnight regulation, liver glucose release, waking demand, stress signaling, sleep quality, and recovery state. A rise during the morning can be part of the system's transition from fasting sleep conditions to daytime demand conditions.

Stress load can further change fasting regulation. Stress signaling may increase the perceived need for accessible fuel. During fasting, when incoming fuel is absent, that perceived need may be met through internal release. Blood sugar can move upward without eating because the system is preserving availability under demand.

This stress-related movement is not a moral failure or evidence that fasting has failed. It is the system interpreting conditions and adjusting supply. The glucose pattern reflects demand-oriented regulation, shaped by counter-regulatory signaling, liver output, tissue uptake, and recovery margin.

Sleep and recovery influence the same process. Sleep disruption can alter signal timing, baseline tendency, counter-regulatory tone, and tissue response. Low recovery capacity can make the system less precise in coordinating internal release with uptake. During fasting, these effects may become more visible because food input is no longer the dominant visible variable.

A well-recovered state may allow fasting regulation to remain more contained. A constrained recovery state may produce more movement, higher morning availability, or slower settling. These differences do not make fasting inherently beneficial or harmful. They show that fasting interacts with the condition of the system receiving it.

Demand also matters. Physical demand, cognitive demand, emotional demand, recovery demand, and environmental demand can all influence how much availability the system preserves. During fasting, the system must meet these demands without incoming fuel. Internal release and counter-regulatory signaling become part of that matching process.

This is why fasting should be understood as context, not proof of control. It changes the regulatory problem. The system must maintain availability while input is reduced, output continues, and demand may change. The result depends on how well internal release, tissue uptake, insulin adjustment, counter-regulatory signaling, and recovery margin coordinate.

Fasting can produce cleaner patterns when internal control is well matched to demand and uptake. It can also expose variability when internal release is prolonged, counter-regulatory signals are strong, tissue uptake is constrained, or baseline tendency is elevated. The fasting state does not impose one outcome. It reveals the system's current capacity for internal regulation.

The Fasting Interaction Mechanism clarifies that blood sugar patterns during fasting are not empty patterns. They are not simply what happens when food is removed. They are active expressions of regulation under reduced input. The system continues to preserve availability, remove glucose, adjust signals, and manage demand.

Blood sugar stability during fasting depends on coordination. Internal release must provide enough availability without becoming excessive. Tissue uptake must continue without drawing availability too low. Insulin signaling must adjust to reduced input while still coordinating storage, uptake, and release. Counter-regulatory signaling must preserve supply without becoming mismatched to demand.

Stability across fasting states therefore depends on regulatory margin. A system with more margin can absorb the absence of input with less volatility. A system with less margin may show greater movement because each internal adjustment carries more effect. Fasting does not create regulation; it reveals how regulation behaves when external input recedes.

This makes fasting neither a shortcut nor a verdict. It is a condition that shifts emphasis from incoming fuel toward internal control. Blood sugar during fasting reflects liver release, tissue uptake, counter-regulatory signaling, insulin adjustment, demand, baseline state, and recovery capacity. Its meaning comes from the interaction of those layers across time.

When food input is absent, blood sugar regulation becomes more visibly dependent on what the system can provide, preserve, remove, and coordinate internally. Fasting interacts with stability by changing the balance of supply and demand, exposing the relationship between internal release, counter-regulation, tissue uptake, and recovery margin.

The next layer is stress, because stress can shift that internal control system even when food input has not changed.

The Stress Interaction Mechanism

Stress can change blood sugar even when food input has not changed, because the system may interpret stress as demand. Blood sugar is not only shaped by what enters from food. It is also shaped by what the body prepares for, responds to, and attempts to support. When the system detects conditions that require readiness, it may preserve or increase glucose availability through internal release, counter-regulatory signaling, altered tissue uptake, and changes in insulin coordination.

The Stress Interaction Mechanism explains this demand-oriented layer of blood sugar regulation. Stress does not have to mean emotional distress alone. It can include physical load, cognitive demand, environmental pressure, sleep disruption, recovery strain, fasting-related demand, workload, illness-like burden, or any condition that increases the system's need to mobilize resources. The common feature is not the subjective label of stress, but the system's interpretation that availability may need to be protected.

This is why stress-related glucose movement can be confusing when blood sugar is interpreted only through food. A person may not have eaten recently, or intake may be unchanged, yet blood sugar may rise or remain elevated. In a food-only model, this appears random. In a regulatory model, the cause may be internal: the system is increasing or preserving accessible fuel because demand signaling has shifted.

Stress-related glucose movement is often misunderstood because it is invisible at the point of origin. A meal is visible. A stress signal is not. Liver glucose release is not directly felt as a discrete event. Counter-regulatory signaling does not announce itself as a simple cause. The visible glucose pattern may therefore be assigned to the wrong source, or interpreted as regulation failing without recognizing that the system is responding to demand.

Demand signaling does not require conscious decision. The body does not wait for deliberate interpretation before altering fuel availability. It can prepare for activity, challenge, vigilance, or strain before actual fuel use becomes obvious. Glucose availability may increase even when physical movement is low, because the system is not only responding to energy already spent. It may also be preparing for energy that might be needed.

This distinction between perceived demand and immediate fuel use is central. The system can mobilize glucose in anticipation of demand, not only as repayment for demand already completed. Stress signaling can shift the system toward readiness, and readiness requires accessible fuel. The resulting blood sugar movement may look disproportionate if interpreted only through visible activity, but it becomes more coherent when understood as preparation.

Glucose availability is therefore different from glucose intake. Blood sugar can rise during stress without new food because the body can add glucose from within. The liver can release glucose into circulation, and counter-regulatory signals can support that release. The pattern is not a contradiction of fasting or absence of food. It is evidence that internal control remains active.

Counter-regulatory signaling provides one pathway through which stress affects blood sugar. These glucose-raising and availability-preserving signals help the system defend access to fuel under demand. Their role is not inherently destabilizing. They allow blood sugar to remain available when the system interprets conditions as requiring support.

The stability question is whether those signals match the demand in timing, proportion, and duration. If stress-related signaling appears briefly and resolves as conditions change, glucose movement may remain contained. If signaling becomes frequent, prolonged, or poorly matched to actual tissue uptake, the pattern may become more elevated, more variable, or slower to settle. The signal remains regulatory, but its fit determines its stability value.

The liver is central to this interaction. During stress, demand-oriented signaling can increase liver glucose release, adding internal supply to circulation. This can happen even when food intake is unchanged or absent. The liver is not acting as a problem organ in this frame. It is functioning as an internal supply layer that responds to signals about need.

When liver release increases under stress, blood sugar may rise because the system is prioritizing availability. The rise is not necessarily tied to a recent meal. It may reflect a state in which the body is preserving access to fuel. This is especially visible when food input is reduced, because internal release becomes easier to identify as a contributor to the pattern.

Insulin signaling remains part of this environment. Stress does not erase insulin regulation, and it does not simply defeat it. Instead, stress changes the coordination problem. Insulin may be signaling uptake and storage, while counter-regulatory signals may be supporting availability and release. The system must negotiate between handling circulating glucose and preserving fuel access for perceived demand.

This competing signal environment can change the blood sugar pattern. If insulin-supported uptake is well matched to tissue demand, glucose released during stress may be used or cleared more smoothly. If availability-preserving signals remain strong while tissue uptake is not proportionate, glucose may stay elevated longer. The pattern reflects coordination among signals rather than the action of one hormone alone.

Tissue uptake determines whether increased availability is matched by removal. If tissues are actively using glucose, stress-related release may be paired with demand. Fuel is made available, and tissues draw from circulation. In that context, the glucose movement may be part of a coordinated demand response.

If demand signaling is high but tissue uptake is lower, slower, or constrained, the pattern changes. The system may increase availability, but tissues may not remove glucose at the same rate. Blood sugar can then remain elevated longer or require more regulatory effort to return toward range. This is a coordination issue, not a moral failure.

Fasting makes the stress interaction more visible. When food input is absent, any glucose movement is less easily explained by incoming fuel. Stress-related counter-regulatory signaling and liver glucose release can become more apparent. Blood sugar may rise during fasting not because fasting has paused regulation, but because fasting has exposed internal control.

This interaction also explains why fasting patterns can differ under different stress states. A fasting interval in a settled recovery state may show one pattern, while a fasting interval under workload, poor sleep, or emotional demand may show another. The absence of food may be the same, but the internal demand environment is not. Fasting removes one input layer while leaving stress signaling, liver release, tissue uptake, and recovery margin in place.

Morning glucose patterns often combine these same forces. The morning transition is not only a time after sleep. It is a shift from overnight regulation into waking demand. The system may increase availability as alertness, movement, and engagement approach. Counter-regulatory signaling, liver glucose release, sleep quality, and stress load can all influence the pattern before food appears.

A morning rise should therefore not be reduced to the previous meal alone. It may reflect overnight regulation, internal release, waking demand, and the recovery state the system carries into the day. Stress load can shape that transition by increasing availability-preserving signals or altering the timing of release and uptake.

Sleep and recovery influence stress-related glucose movement because they affect regulatory margin. When recovery is sufficient, signals may resolve more cleanly, tissue response may be more coordinated, and the system may settle more efficiently after demand. When recovery is limited, demand signaling may become more prominent, and the same stress load may produce greater glucose movement.

Sleep disruption can alter timing. Internal release may occur differently, counter-regulatory signaling may be more active, and insulin coordination may become less precise. The result can be a more reactive glucose pattern, especially during morning transition or fasting states. This does not turn sleep into a moral category. It shows that recovery state changes the conditions under which regulation operates.

Repeated stress signaling can contribute to baseline elevation. If the system frequently interprets conditions as demand, availability preservation may become more persistent. Liver glucose release may remain more active, and counter-regulatory tone may become more prominent. Over time, the ordinary return point can drift upward or require greater effort to maintain.

This upward shift is not caused by stress as a single event. It develops through repetition, duration, and context. A short demand state may produce a temporary movement. Repeated or unresolved demand signaling can change the baseline environment. The system may spend more time preserving availability and less time in a settled return state.

Stress can also amplify variability. Demand-oriented signaling may create more frequent glucose movement, especially when combined with constrained tissue uptake, reduced recovery, fasting exposure, or elevated baseline tendency. A stress-related rise may be followed by stronger correction. A correction may be followed by counter-regulatory rebound.

Movement becomes wider or slower to resolve when regulatory margin is reduced.

Variability under stress reflects the interaction between readiness and recovery. The system may prepare fuel repeatedly, then attempt to clear or settle that availability afterward. If the signals do not resolve smoothly, blood sugar movement can become more reactive. The pattern is still regulatory, but regulation is operating under greater effort.

The Stress Interaction Mechanism changes interpretation by separating stress-related glucose movement from blame. A rise during stress is not a character statement. It is not evidence of weakness, poor coping, or emotional failure. It is a demand-response pattern in which the body adjusts availability according to perceived or actual need.

This does not mean every glucose movement during stress is automatically stable. A response can be understandable and still become prolonged, mismatched, or effortful. The mechanism explains why the movement occurs; it also shows why coordination matters. Stability depends on whether release, uptake, insulin signaling, counter-regulation, and recovery margin remain matched to the demand.

Stress-related blood sugar movement is therefore neither random nor purely food-driven. It reflects the system's attempt to maintain readiness and preserve access to fuel. The visible pattern may include rising glucose, prolonged elevation, slower recovery, or wider variability, but the underlying logic is demand-oriented regulation.

Blood sugar stability depends on how stress signaling is integrated with the rest of the system. Internal release must match need. Tissue uptake must match availability. Insulin signaling must coordinate handling without ignoring preservation. Counter-regulatory signaling must support demand without remaining stronger than the situation requires. Baseline tendency and recovery margin shape how cleanly these transitions occur.

As stress load interacts with fasting state, morning transition, tissue demand, and prior conditions, blood sugar becomes an expression of more than intake. It becomes a visible output of the system's readiness logic. Stress can raise glucose availability because the body may be preparing for demand, not because regulation has disappeared.

The stability question is not whether stress signals exist, but whether the system can settle after demand. Blood sugar regulation requires the ability to mobilize fuel and then return toward range as conditions change. That return depends heavily on sleep and recovery, because recovery shapes signal timing, regulatory margin, baseline tendency, and the system's ability to settle after demand.

The Sleep Interaction Mechanism

Sleep affects blood sugar regulation not by acting as a single lever, but by changing the recovery and timing environment in which regulation occurs. Blood sugar does not move through a timeless system. It is shaped by daily rhythms, recovery state, signal timing, tissue response, internal release, and the transition between rest and waking demand. Sleep influences these conditions together, which is why its effect on blood sugar cannot be reduced to one isolated pathway.

The Sleep Interaction Mechanism explains sleep as part of the regulatory environment. Sleep and recovery help shape how precisely signals are timed, how tissues respond to glucose availability, how internal release is coordinated overnight, and how the system returns toward range after demand. Sleep is not a behavioral grade. It is one of the conditions that determines how much margin the system has for regulation.

Sleep-related glucose patterns are often misunderstood because they appear at a distance from obvious causes. A morning glucose pattern may be attributed to prior food, stress alone, random variation, or personal discipline. Those explanations can miss the timing environment beneath the visible number. Morning blood sugar can reflect overnight regulation, liver glucose release, counter-regulatory signaling, insulin response, tissue uptake, sleep state, and recovery capacity.

Sleep matters not only as a period of time but as the recovery state carried forward into the next cycle. Recovery capacity influences how cleanly the system settles after demand and how prepared it is for the next regulatory challenge. A system that has recovered more fully may have more room to coordinate input, fasting, stress, and morning transition without excessive effort. A constrained recovery state may leave less margin for the same conditions.

Regulatory margin is the space available for adjustment before movement becomes larger, slower, or more reactive. When recovery capacity is stronger, the system can often absorb ordinary variation with less visible disruption. Signals may rise and resolve more cleanly. Tissue uptake may align more effectively with availability. Internal release may support need without remaining more active than the situation requires.

When recovery is constrained, the same regulatory events can become more effortful. A fasting interval, waking transition, stress load, or ordinary demand state may produce larger or slower glucose movement because the system has less margin. The issue is not that regulation has disappeared. It is that regulation must operate with reduced capacity for clean timing and resolution.

Circadian timing adds another layer. Blood sugar regulation includes processes that follow temporal organization: internal release, insulin response, tissue uptake, counter-regulatory signaling, and morning transition. These processes do not occur in an undifferentiated background. The system's readiness to release, store, use, or preserve fuel changes across time, and sleep is part of that timing structure.

Circadian timing does not act as a simple switch. It organizes the background conditions under which signals become more or less prominent. A glucose-raising signal at one point in the cycle may have a different effect than the same signal under a different recovery state or transition period. Timing changes the context in which release, uptake, and insulin response are interpreted.

This is why blood sugar regulation cannot be fully understood as if every hour were metabolically identical. The system is always regulating, but it is not regulating from the same timing environment at every point in the day. Sleep helps shape that environment by influencing when the system is recovering, when it is maintaining availability, and when it is preparing to meet waking demand.

Signal timing affects interpretation. A glucose pattern that appears in the morning is not only a delayed report on what entered the system before sleep. It may be produced by the shift from overnight maintenance toward waking demand. Internal release, counter-regulatory tone, insulin response, and tissue uptake can all change as the body moves from rest into activity readiness. The pattern belongs to a transition, not a single cause.

Insulin signaling is shaped by this recovery and timing environment. Insulin helps coordinate uptake, storage, and reduced internal release when glucose availability changes. Sleep and recovery can influence how precisely that signal aligns with tissue response and current demand. This does not mean insulin is defeated by poor sleep or perfected by good sleep. It means signal interpretation occurs within a system state.

When recovery is stronger, insulin-supported coordination may occur with less regulatory strain. Tissues may receive and use signals in a more settled environment, and internal release may adjust more cleanly. When recovery is constrained, the same signal may operate in a system carrying more stress-state signaling, less margin, or altered baseline tendency. The visible blood sugar pattern reflects that broader environment.

Overnight regulation depends heavily on internal release. During sleep, external food input is usually absent for an extended period, yet tissues continue using glucose. The liver can release glucose to preserve availability across this interval. This release is not an abnormal interruption of sleep. It is part of maintaining blood sugar as a regulated variable when incoming fuel is not present.

Morning glucose patterns can reflect the balance of this overnight regulation. If internal release, tissue uptake, and counter-regulatory signaling remain coordinated, the transition may appear contained. If release is more active, uptake is slower, stress signaling is stronger, or recovery margin is reduced, the morning pattern may appear higher or more variable. The number is a surface expression of multiple overnight processes.

Counter-regulatory signaling also participates in the sleep-wake transition. As waking approaches, the system may preserve or increase glucose availability to support alertness, movement, and engagement. This availability support can occur before food is eaten. Morning glucose can therefore reflect readiness signaling as much as intake history.

This makes morning glucose especially easy to overinterpret. The number appears at a clean point in the day, before new food has entered, so it may seem like a simple baseline. But it can contain the residue of overnight regulation, the transition into waking demand, the level of recovery available, and the strength of stress-state signaling. It is a morning value, but it is not produced by one morning cause.

A higher or more variable morning pattern therefore belongs to a broader timing and recovery environment. It may show how internal release, counter-regulation, insulin response, and tissue uptake coordinated across the night and into waking. The value is visible in the morning, but the mechanism begins earlier.

Stress load overlaps with sleep in this mechanism. Stress-state signaling can increase availability pressure, while sleep and recovery shape how well that pressure resolves. If stress load remains elevated into the night or recovery is limited, the system may carry demand-oriented signaling into overnight regulation and morning transition. Blood sugar movement may then become more reactive, prolonged, or elevated at the start of the day.

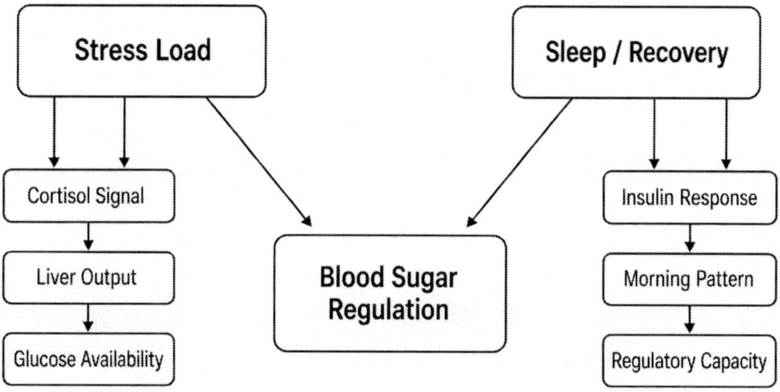

[Figure 9: Stress and Sleep Influence]

The figure matters because stress and sleep influence blood sugar regulation through overlapping but different pathways. Stress load can increase availability pressure through demand-oriented signaling, liver output, and glucose availability. Sleep and recovery shape the system's ability to respond to that pressure through insulin response, morning pattern, and regulatory capacity. One side increases the demand to mobilize; the other shapes the capacity to coordinate and settle.

This distinction helps explain why the same stress signal can produce different blood sugar patterns in different recovery states. Under stronger recovery, the system may absorb demand signaling with less visible disturbance. Under constrained recovery, the same pressure may lead to greater internal release, slower settling, or a more elevated morning pattern.

Tissue uptake is also influenced by recovery state. Tissues continue using glucose overnight and into the morning, but the rate and coordination of uptake depend on demand, signaling, and capacity. Recovery processes themselves require energy, and ordinary cellular work continues during rest. The visible blood sugar level reflects both what the liver releases and what tissues remove.

When uptake is well matched to release, glucose availability can remain more contained. When uptake is constrained or signaling coordination is less precise, internal release may exceed removal for longer periods. This does not mean the system is inactive. It means the balance between output and internal supply has shifted under the influence of recovery state and timing.

Sleep and fasting often overlap. Overnight is commonly a fasting interval, and that overlap can make internal control more visible. Food input is absent, but internal release, tissue uptake, counter-regulation, and insulin adjustment continue. Morning patterns emerge from that interaction. They are not simply reports on the last meal or signs that nothing occurred overnight.

This overlap helps explain why sleep disruption can change fasting patterns. With reduced recovery, the system may rely more heavily on availability-preserving signals. Internal release may be more active, tissue response may differ, and the return toward baseline may take longer. The fasting state exposes the internal side of regulation, while sleep quality shapes the precision of that regulation.

Repeated poor recovery can contribute to baseline elevation. If the system often enters the morning with stronger internal release, higher stress-state signaling, constrained tissue uptake, or slower signal resolution, the ordinary return point may drift upward. Baseline elevation is not a single morning event. It is a time-based pattern in which the resting tendency becomes more effortful or less settled.

This upward drift reflects accumulated regulation, not a moral failure. The system may still be correcting, clearing, releasing, and preserving availability. But if recovery is insufficient for clean resolution, regulation may begin from a higher or more constrained baseline. The next input, stressor, or fasting interval then enters that altered state.

Sleep disruption can also contribute to variability amplification. When recovery is constrained, glucose movement may become larger, more frequent, or slower to settle. A morning rise may take longer to resolve. A stress-related release may produce wider movement. A correction may overshoot more easily because signal timing is less precise. Variability increases when the system has less margin for clean adjustment.

The important distinction is that sleep-related variability is not the same as failure of regulation. It may reflect regulation working harder under reduced recovery. Internal release may be attempting to preserve availability. Insulin signaling may be attempting to coordinate uptake. Counter-regulatory signals may be supporting demand. The pattern becomes less contained because these layers are operating with less recovery margin.

The Sleep Interaction Mechanism changes interpretation by shifting attention from single causes to coordination. A morning pattern is not simply a food report. It is not simply a stress report. It is not a grade on sleep behavior. It is an expression of overnight regulation, internal release, tissue uptake, counter-regulation, insulin response, baseline tendency, and recovery capacity.

This interpretation also prevents sleep from becoming a moral category. Poor sleep, disrupted sleep, or limited recovery should not be read as personal failure within blood sugar regulation. They are system conditions. They alter the regulatory environment by changing timing, margin, demand signaling, and the ability to settle after demand.

Blood sugar stability depends on the system's ability to coordinate across these layers. It must preserve availability overnight without excessive release. It must support tissue uptake while food input is absent. It must adjust insulin signaling and counter-regulation as the body moves toward waking demand. It must return toward range after stress and settle into a baseline that remains workable across time.

Sleep and recovery shape that ability to settle. They influence whether signals resolve, whether internal release tapers, whether tissue uptake aligns with demand, and whether variability remains contained. Blood sugar stability therefore depends on integrating multiple layers of regulation rather than isolating one variable and treating it as the whole system.

The Integration Mechanism

Blood sugar stability is not produced by one layer of regulation, but by the interaction of many layers at once. Food input matters, but it is not the whole pattern. Tissue uptake matters, but it does not operate apart from supply. Liver glucose release matters, but it responds to signals, demand, and context. Insulin and counter-regulatory signals matter, but neither side explains stability alone.

The Integration Mechanism explains blood sugar as the visible result of coordinated layers operating across time. Incoming fuel, tissue output, internal release, insulin signaling, counter-regulation, stress load, sleep and recovery, fasting state, activity demand, baseline tendency, correction, variability, and regulatory margin all shape the final pattern. Integration is not addition. It is interaction. Each layer changes the meaning and effect of the others.

Blood sugar is commonly misunderstood because visible patterns invite single-cause explanations. A rise may be assigned to food. A morning pattern may be assigned to the prior meal. A fasting rise may appear unexplained. A stress-related elevation may seem random. A sharp decline may be interpreted as a personal weakness or behavioral problem. These interpretations isolate one visible feature while excluding the system state that produced it.

Isolation simplifies the pattern, but it also removes the relationships that make the pattern understandable. Food does not act on an empty system. Stress does not act on an empty system. Sleep disruption does not act on an empty system. Fasting does not occur in a neutral background. Each layer arrives into a system that already has a baseline, a margin, a recovery state, a demand state, and a recent regulatory history.

This is why the same visible trigger can produce different blood sugar patterns across different contexts. The trigger may be similar, but the receiving system is not identical. Integration explains why the question cannot stop at what entered the system or what signal appeared. It must also include the state of the system receiving that input or signal.

Food input and tissue output show why isolation fails. Food introduces fuel into circulation, but the blood sugar response depends on what tissues remove, use, store, or redirect. Input has no complete meaning without output. A meal entering a system with higher tissue demand is not handled the same way as the same meal entering a system with constrained uptake or low recovery capacity.

The reverse is also true. Tissue output cannot be understood without supply. Tissues remove glucose from circulation, but what they remove depends on what has entered from food, what the liver is releasing, and what signals are coordinating storage and use. Blood sugar reflects the relationship between appearance and removal, not either process alone.

Liver release adds a second supply path. Glucose can enter circulation from food, but it can also enter from within the body. During fasting, morning transition, stress, or demand states, internal release may preserve availability even when food input is absent. This means blood sugar is not simply a report on eating. It is a report on total supply and total removal.

Incoming fuel and liver release can overlap. A meal may arrive while internal release is still active. A stress signal may increase release even when recent food has not changed. A fasting state may show movement because the liver is maintaining availability. Integration means recognizing that supply does not come from one source.

Insulin signaling and counter-regulatory signaling form another paired layer. Insulin helps coordinate uptake, storage, and reduced internal release when fuel is available. Counter-regulatory signals help preserve or raise availability when supply is needed. These signals move in different directions, but they belong to the same control system.

Stability depends on their timing and proportion. If glucose-lowering signals match incoming fuel and tissue demand, movement can resolve cleanly. If availability-preserving signals match fasting, stress, or demand, internal release can support function. If either side arrives too late, lasts too long, or exceeds the need, movement can become prolonged, reactive, or unstable.

Fed and fasting states shift the emphasis of regulation. In a fed state, incoming fuel handling becomes more visible. The system must distribute, store, and clear what enters. In a fasting state, internal control becomes more visible. The system must maintain availability through liver release, counter-regulation, insulin adjustment, and tissue uptake while food input is absent.

Neither state is inherently superior as a regulatory concept. Each changes the coordination problem. The fed state emphasizes integration of incoming supply. The fasting state emphasizes internal maintenance. Stability depends on the system's ability to move between these states without losing coordination.

Stress load changes the system by increasing availability pressure. When stress is interpreted as demand, the body may preserve or raise glucose availability through counter-regulatory signaling and liver release. This can occur even without new food input. Stress-related movement is not random; it reflects demand-oriented regulation.

Stress also interacts with fasting and baseline tendency. A fasting interval under low stress and adequate recovery may look different from a fasting interval under high demand. A system with an elevated baseline may respond differently to the same stress signal than one with more regulatory margin. The stress layer changes other layers rather than acting alone.

Sleep and recovery shape the ability to settle. Recovery capacity influences signal timing, tissue response, internal release, morning transition, and regulatory margin. When recovery is stronger, the system may return toward range with less effort. When recovery is constrained, the same input, stress signal, or fasting interval may produce larger or slower movement.

Circadian timing adds structure to this interaction. Morning patterns can reflect overnight fasting, liver release, counter-regulation, insulin response, waking demand, and sleep state. A morning reading is not merely a delayed food report. It is the surface of overnight and early-day coordination.

Activity demand changes output. When tissues require more fuel, glucose uptake may be different than when demand is lower. Activity in this framework is not advice or a prescription. It is a demand state. It changes how much glucose tissues may remove and how supply is interpreted.

When demand and availability align, glucose movement may resolve differently than when availability rises without proportionate uptake. If the liver releases glucose for demand and tissues use it, the pattern may be contained. If availability rises while uptake is constrained, glucose may remain elevated longer. Integration depends on matching supply to removal.

Baseline tendency determines the ordinary return point. Variability describes movement around that point. A system can fluctuate and still remain stable if it returns toward a settled range. If baseline drifts upward, each new movement begins from a more effortful starting point. If variability amplifies, movement becomes wider, more frequent, or slower to recover.

These two patterns interact. A higher baseline reduces margin for additional movement. Amplified variability makes return less predictable. Together, they can make regulation more effortful even when the system is still actively correcting. Instability is not the absence of regulation. It is regulation working with reduced containment.

Correction is necessary, but correction must be integrated. Glucose-lowering forces respond to excess availability. Glucose-raising forces respond to threatened availability. When these responses fit the need, they restore range. When they overshoot, they can create counter-correction, rebound, and oscillation.

Overcorrection shows why more force is not the same as more stability. A strong response can move beyond the intended range. A delayed response can create a larger correction than would have been needed earlier. A prolonged response can continue after conditions have changed. Integration requires correction that resolves, not correction that creates the next disruption.

Timing and proportion organize every layer. Food appearance has timing. Tissue uptake has timing. Liver release has timing. Insulin signaling and counter-regulation have timing. Stress and sleep influence timing. Fasting changes timing by removing external input. Stability depends on whether these signals appear, scale, and resolve in relation to current demand.

Proportion determines whether a response fits the situation. Too little clearance may prolong elevation. Too much clearance may threaten availability. Too little release may leave supply unsupported. Too much release may extend glucose movement beyond demand. The system does not need one side to dominate. It needs each response to match context.

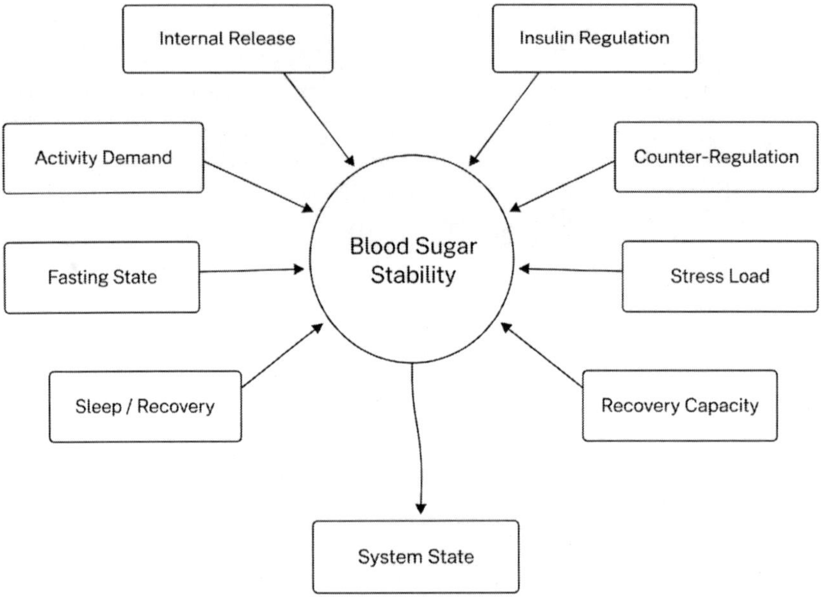

Stability emerges from coordination, not one isolated variable.

[Figure 10: Full Blood Sugar Stability System]

The figure matters because it places the visible blood sugar pattern at the center of interacting forces rather than at the end of a single cause. Food input, tissue output, liver release, insulin regulation, counter-regulation, stress load, sleep and recovery, fasting state, activity demand, and recovery capacity all feed into the same stability problem. None of these layers is separate from the others once regulation is underway.

The feedback arrow is equally important. Blood sugar stability is not only an outcome of system state; it also becomes part of the next system state. A prolonged elevation, sharp decline, rebound, or slower recovery can change the conditions under which the next input, fasting interval, stress signal, or demand state is handled. The system is continuously receiving the consequences of its own prior regulation.

Regulatory margin determines how much disturbance the system can absorb before movement becomes excessive, prolonged, or unstable. A system with more margin can handle input, fasting, stress, sleep disruption, activity demand, and internal release with less visible volatility. A system with less margin may show larger movement from the same conditions.

Constraint narrows margin. Stress load, poor recovery, reduced tissue uptake, repeated overcorrection, baseline elevation, and persistent internal release can all reduce the space available for clean adjustment. Under constraint, ordinary events become more consequential because the system has less room to buffer them.

Integration changes interpretation. The useful question is not simply what caused a number. A visible blood sugar pattern is rarely the product of one layer alone. The more complete question is which layers are interacting in the pattern: input, output, liver release, insulin signaling, counter-regulation, stress load, sleep and recovery, fasting state, activity demand, baseline tendency, variability, and margin.

This does not make interpretation vague. It makes it more accurate. A rise after food still includes food. A fasting rise still includes internal release. A stress-related movement still includes demand signaling. A morning pattern still includes overnight regulation. The point is not to erase causes, but to place each cause inside the system that gives it meaning.

This prepares the ground for the next mechanism: constraint. Integration explains how the layers interact; constraint explains where coordination becomes harder to maintain. A system can integrate many signals well when margin is broad, timing is clean, and recovery is sufficient. The same system may struggle when margin narrows, timing becomes mismatched, or repeated demand reduces the room for correction.

Constraint does not mean the system stops regulating. It means regulation occurs within tighter boundaries. The next chapter moves from the interaction of layers to the limits within which those layers can remain coordinated.

The Integration Mechanism brings the regulatory model together. Blood sugar stability emerges when food input, tissue uptake, internal release, insulin signaling, counter-regulation, fasting state, stress load, sleep and recovery, activity demand, baseline tendency, correction, and margin remain coordinated enough for movement to stay contained and recoverable.

Every visible pattern is the surface of this coordination. Blood sugar does not simply report what was eaten, how much insulin appeared, whether fasting occurred, or whether stress was present. It reports the interaction of supply, demand, signaling, recovery, timing, and constraint. Every system has limits, and blood sugar stability depends on the range within which those layers can remain coordinated.

The Constraint Mechanism

Blood sugar regulation has limits, and those limits shape how much disturbance the system can absorb before movement becomes wider, slower, or more effortful. The body can correct, compensate, release, clear, store, preserve availability, and recover, but none of those processes operate with infinite capacity. Every layer of regulation depends on available margin.

The Constraint Mechanism explains what happens when that margin narrows. Constraint does not mean blood sugar regulation has stopped. It means regulation is operating with less room to absorb disturbance cleanly. The same meal, fasting interval, stress load, sleep disruption, activity demand, morning transition, or internal release pattern can produce a different glucose response when the system has less buffer.

A constrained system may still regulate continuously. It can still move glucose into tissues, release glucose from the liver, adjust insulin signaling, activate counter-regulatory support, and return toward range. The difference is not the presence or absence of regulation. The difference is the cost, speed, precision, and containment of that regulation.

Constraint is often misread as failure because the visible pattern becomes harder to interpret. A larger rise may look like a food problem. A slower return may look like broken regulation. A fasting increase may look random. A morning elevation may be assigned to the prior meal. These interpretations isolate the visible movement while missing the reduced margin underneath it.

Constraint is better understood as a systems condition. It can reflect reduced buffer, higher demand, slower recovery, altered timing, narrower adaptive reserve, lower tissue uptake capacity, or accumulated regulatory load. None of these is a moral category. They describe the conditions under which regulation must operate.

Compensation is one way the system preserves function under constraint. When demand increases or margin narrows, the system can signal more strongly, release more glucose internally, preserve availability more often, correct more aggressively, or extend recovery efforts across a longer period. Compensation allows function to continue even when conditions are less favorable.

But compensation uses margin. A system that repeatedly compensates has less room available for the next disturbance. If internal release is more active, if counter-regulatory tone remains elevated, if insulin signaling must work harder to coordinate uptake, or if tissue clearance is slower, the system may still remain functional while accumulating regulatory cost.

Compensation can hide constraint for a time. The visible pattern may appear managed because blood sugar still returns toward range, but the return may require more effort than before. Over time, the system may spend less time settled and more time correcting, preserving, rebounding, or recovering. The apparent stability becomes more expensive.

Chronic stress narrows margin by keeping demand-oriented signaling more active. When the system repeatedly interprets conditions as requiring readiness, it may preserve more glucose availability through counter-regulatory signaling and liver glucose release. This can raise the background pressure on blood sugar regulation even when food input has not changed.

Stress-related constraint is not simply a momentary rise. It can change the system's operating environment. If demand signaling remains frequent or prolonged, the system spends more time in availability-preservation mode and less time in settled return. Internal release may be more active, baseline tendency may drift upward, and variability may become easier to amplify.

Poor sleep and disrupted recovery narrow margin from another direction. Recovery helps signals resolve, tissue uptake coordinate, internal release taper, and the system settle after demand. When recovery is limited, new regulatory challenges may arrive before earlier adjustments have fully completed.

This overlap changes the next response. A meal may arrive into a system still carrying stress-state signaling. A fasting interval may begin from a baseline that has not fully settled. A morning transition may occur after overnight regulation that was more effortful than usual. The same event then produces a different blood sugar pattern because the system did not begin from the same state.

Aging can also change margin, but it should not be interpreted as collapse. Aging may alter adaptive reserve, recovery speed, tissue responsiveness, muscle buffer, and tolerance for repeated volatility. These changes do not erase regulation. They change the amount of regulatory room available for absorbing disturbance and returning cleanly toward range.

Adaptive reserve is the capacity to absorb change without requiring disproportionate compensation. When reserve narrows, smaller challenges can become more consequential. A stress signal, sleep disruption, fasting interval, or glucose appearance that once required modest adjustment may require more effort under lower reserve. The system still responds, but the response may be slower or less contained.

Low recovery capacity can appear across contexts, not only through sleep or age. It can reflect accumulated demand, illness burden, repeated volatility, high stress load, incomplete repair, or overlapping regulatory demands. In this state, the system enters new challenges before previous regulation has fully resolved.

This creates layering. Output may still be adjusting while internal release increases. Counter-regulatory signaling may still be active while insulin-supported uptake is needed. Tissue demand may shift before baseline has settled. Regulation becomes more complex because the system is not handling one clean event at a time.

Reduced muscle buffer constrains regulation through the tissue side of blood sugar control. Muscle acts as a major tissue sink for glucose use and storage. It helps create room for glucose movement by drawing fuel from circulation and holding some of that fuel for later availability. When that buffer is smaller, less responsive, or less demanded, glucose removal may become less efficient.

This does not make muscle mass a moral measure or activity level a character statement. It simply describes a regulatory layer. Tissue uptake is one way the system clears glucose. When the available tissue sink is reduced or demand is lower, the same glucose availability may remain in circulation longer or require more signaling effort to move into storage and use.

Illness burden or inflammatory burden can narrow margin by creating competing demand. The system may be coordinating defense, repair, altered signaling, internal release, tissue uptake, and recovery at the same time. Blood sugar regulation does not stop during these states, but it operates alongside other priorities.

Competing demand changes interpretation. A glucose pattern during physiological strain may reflect more than food input or fasting duration. It may reflect internal release supporting demand, counter-regulatory signaling preserving availability, tissue uptake shifting under strain, and recovery capacity being allocated elsewhere. The system is still regulating, but it is regulating inside a more crowded environment.

Repeated volatility becomes a constraint because every swing requires response. Wider movement, sharper declines, rebounds, prolonged elevations, and oscillations all consume regulatory effort. The more time the system spends correcting, the less time it spends settled.

Volatility also changes the starting point for future regulation. A rebound can become the background for the next correction. A prolonged elevation can become the starting state for the next input. A sharp decline can trigger availability defense. Each movement creates another demand for response, and the system begins to operate within accumulated motion rather than settled range.

Baseline elevation narrows margin by raising the ordinary starting point. When the system's return point drifts upward, new disturbances begin from a more effortful baseline. A meal, stress signal, fasting interval, morning transition, or activity demand has less room before movement becomes prolonged or harder to resolve.

Baseline elevation and variability often reinforce each other. A higher baseline leaves less room for additional movement, and wider variability makes return less consistent. Together, they reduce containment. The system may still correct each movement, but the return point remains less settled and the next movement begins with less margin.

Overcorrection adds another cost. A response meant to restore range can overshoot, creating the need for counter-correction. A strong lowering response can produce a decline that triggers glucose-raising signals. A rebound can then require further correction. Regulation remains present, but the system becomes more active because each correction creates another problem to resolve.

Oscillation is expensive because it keeps the system moving. Instead of a rise resolving cleanly, the system alternates between lowering and raising forces. Insulin-supported uptake, counter-regulatory signaling, liver release, tissue uptake, and availability defense may all participate. The issue is not that any one signal is wrong; it is that timing and proportion have become costly.

The same challenge can therefore produce different patterns depending on current capacity. The same meal may be handled smoothly after stronger recovery and more effortfully after poor sleep or stress load. The food input is similar, but the receiving system has changed. Tissue uptake, liver release, insulin coordination, and regulatory margin are not the same.

The same fasting interval can also produce different responses. In one state, internal release and tissue uptake may remain balanced. In another, stress load may increase availability-preserving signaling, or baseline elevation may make the fasting pattern start higher. Food is absent in both cases, but the internal regulatory environment differs.

The same morning transition can vary according to sleep state. Overnight regulation may settle cleanly after stronger recovery, or it may carry forward more counter-regulatory tone after disrupted sleep. Morning glucose then reflects not only the transition into waking demand, but also the recovery state behind that transition.

The same activity demand can produce different glucose patterns depending on tissue sink capacity and prior state. If tissues are ready to receive and use glucose, availability may be matched by uptake. If tissue uptake is constrained or recovery is incomplete, the same demand may require more internal release or produce a slower return toward range.

The same stress signal can also land differently depending on baseline tendency. A system starting from a settled range has more room to absorb availability pressure. A system already elevated or variable has less margin. Stress then becomes more likely to produce a larger or longer-lasting visible movement.

Regulatory margin is the practical space within which the system can adjust without excessive movement. It is not a fixed number. It is the available room for input, output, internal release, insulin signaling, counter-regulation, recovery, and demand to interact without becoming prolonged, exaggerated, or difficult to resolve.

When margin is wider, the system can absorb disturbances with less visible volatility. When margin narrows, ordinary events become more consequential. The system may still respond correctly, but the response may require more time, stronger signals, or additional counter-correction. Constraint narrows the space in which regulation can remain clean.

Constraint accumulation is often more important than any single constraint alone. Stress load, poor recovery, reduced tissue uptake, baseline elevation, illness burden, persistent internal release, repeated volatility, and overcorrection may each be modest in isolation. Together, they reduce the system's ability to absorb new movement.

This accumulation explains why instability can appear gradually. No single event may seem large enough to explain the pattern. Yet the system may be carrying multiple small loads at once: incomplete recovery, elevated baseline, stress-state signaling, slower tissue uptake, and repeated correction. The visible glucose movement reflects the combined pressure.

Constraint changes interpretation by replacing blame with capacity analysis. A larger rise is not automatically a food problem. A slower return is not automatically absence of regulation. A fasting rise is not automatically random. A morning elevation is not automatically explained by the prior meal. Each pattern may reflect the system operating with less room for coordination.

The Constraint Mechanism keeps blood sugar stability grounded in limits. Stability depends not only on whether regulatory signals exist, but whether the system has enough buffer, recovery capacity, tissue sink capacity, timing precision, adaptive reserve, and regulatory margin to use those signals cleanly across time.

Blood sugar stability is not judgment or perfection. It is the ability of a constrained regulatory system to maintain coordination across changing conditions. The final framing shifts from what regulation does to how blood sugar patterns should be interpreted without moralizing, over-isolating, or mistaking movement for failure.

The Stability Framing Mechanism

Blood sugar stability is not a single reading, a perfect line, or a micromanaged target. It is coordinated fuel regulation over time. The visible number matters, but it is not the system itself. It is one point on the surface of ongoing regulation, produced by input, output, internal release, signaling, demand, recovery, timing, and constraint.

The Stability Framing Mechanism explains how blood sugar should be interpreted as a regulated process rather than an isolated value. Stability does not mean motionless glucose. It does not mean a spike-free pattern, a permanently flat curve, or a number held in place by direct control. Stability means the system can respond to changing conditions while keeping movement contained, interpretable, and recoverable.

This reframing is necessary because blood sugar is easy to compress into a single visible measurement. A reading feels clear because it is precise. It appears objective because it can be counted. It feels immediate because it belongs to a specific moment. But precision should not be mistaken for completeness. A single value can be accurate and still incomplete as an explanation.

This is the difference between measurement and interpretation. Measurement identifies a point. Interpretation explains what that point belongs to. A blood sugar reading can show where glucose availability was at one moment, but it cannot by itself show how the system arrived there, how much effort was required, whether movement was resolving, or what pressures were shaping the background state.

A number can therefore be useful without being final. It can be part of the evidence without becoming the whole explanation. The mistake is not noticing the number. The mistake is asking the number to carry more meaning than one point in a moving regulatory system can hold.

A reading may reflect food input, tissue uptake, liver glucose release, insulin signaling, counter-regulatory signaling, stress load, fasting state, sleep and recovery, activity demand, baseline tendency, and prior regulatory history. The number is real, but it is not self-explanatory. It is a surface point within a moving sequence.

The appeal of single-reading interpretation is that it reduces complexity. It asks what caused the number and searches for a nearby event. A meal, a fast, a stressful morning, a night of poor sleep, or a period of activity may become the whole explanation. Each may matter, but none automatically explains the entire pattern alone.

A flat-line ideal creates another framing error. Blood sugar is supposed to move because the body is constantly using, storing, releasing, and preserving fuel. Fuel enters. Tissues remove it. The liver releases it. Signals coordinate uptake and storage. Stress and fasting may increase availability. Sleep and recovery shape return. Movement is not evidence that stability is absent.

A perfectly motionless pattern would not represent the full reality of fuel regulation. The body must adapt to fed states, fasting states, stress states, waking transitions, tissue demand, recovery demands, and changing internal supply. Stability is not the refusal to move. It is the ability to move without losing coordination.

A flat-line ideal also hides the purpose of blood sugar movement. Fuel regulation exists because the system has changing needs. Tissues do not demand the same amount of energy at every moment. Food does not enter continuously at the same rate. Internal release does not remain identical across sleep, fasting, stress, and waking transition. A living system cannot be understood as if stillness were the highest form of order.

Order in this system is dynamic. It appears as matched response, appropriate timing, sufficient return, and preserved availability. Stability is not found in the absence of change, but in the system's ability to let change occur without letting that change become disorganized, prolonged, or self-reinforcing.

The difference between movement and instability is therefore central. Movement can reflect ordinary regulation. Blood sugar may rise after input because fuel has entered circulation. It may decline as tissues take up glucose. It may rise during fasting because internal release is preserving availability. It may shift in the morning because the system is moving from overnight regulation into waking demand.

Instability appears when movement becomes excessive, prolonged, poorly matched, difficult to resolve, or repeatedly amplified. The issue is not that glucose rises or falls. The issue is whether the movement fits context, resolves appropriately, returns toward a workable range, and does not create repeated overcorrection or rebound.

Spike-focused interpretation narrows this distinction. A rise becomes the central event, and the question becomes whether the rise occurred. That framing can miss the regulatory context. A rise after input may be expected. A rise during stress may reflect availability preservation. A rise during fasting may reflect internal release. A morning rise may reflect transition rather than recent food alone.

Regulatory framing asks a different question. It does not isolate the rise as a verdict. It asks what system state produced the movement and whether that movement remained contained and recoverable. It considers timing, proportion, demand, baseline tendency, tissue uptake, internal release, and recovery margin.

Target framing creates a related distortion. When blood sugar is treated as a number to micromanage, each movement can appear as a problem to correct. But the system does not regulate by obeying one fixed target. It operates through feedback loops, working ranges, signal timing, tissue response, internal release, and counter-regulation.

Correction is not a sign that regulation has failed. Correction is regulation. The system must correct after input, preserve availability during absence, respond to stress, adjust to demand, and settle after movement. Stability depends on correction that fits the situation, not on the absence of correction.

Judgment framing is the most distorting form of interpretation. Blood sugar movement can become attached to discipline, food virtue, stress failure, sleep failure, body judgment, or personal control. This framing assigns moral meaning to a regulatory output. It treats the surface pattern as a character statement.

Blood sugar movement is not a character statement. It is a signal output of regulation. It reflects the interaction between supply, demand, signaling, recovery, timing, and constraint. Moral language does not clarify the mechanism. It obscures the system producing the pattern.

The stronger frame is coordinated fuel regulation over time. Blood sugar stability means the system can coordinate incoming fuel, tissue uptake, liver glucose release, insulin signaling, counter-regulation, fasting state, stress load, sleep and recovery, activity demand, baseline tendency, variability, correction, and regulatory margin across changing conditions.

Food input becomes one layer rather than the whole explanation. Tissue output gives input its meaning by determining how much glucose is removed, used, stored, or redistributed. Liver glucose release adds internal supply when food is absent or demand increases. Insulin signaling helps coordinate uptake and storage. Counter-regulatory signaling preserves availability when supply needs support.

Stress load changes availability pressure. Sleep and recovery shape timing, margin, and the ability to settle. Fasting reduces incoming fuel and makes internal control more visible. Activity demand changes tissue uptake. Baseline tendency defines the ordinary return point. Variability shows how widely and how often the system moves around that point.

Time scale matters because stability is not fully visible in one moment. A single reading belongs to a larger sequence. Minutes may show a rise or decline. Hours may show recovery or prolonged movement. Days may show baseline tendency, repeated volatility, morning transition, or accumulated regulatory effort. Stability is a time-based property.

This time scale protects the reader from overreacting to isolated movement while still allowing patterns to matter. One movement may not define the system, but repeated movement can reveal how the system is operating. One return may look clean, while repeated returns may begin from a gradually higher baseline. One correction may resolve, while repeated corrections may show that the system is spending more time working than settling.

Blood sugar stability therefore lives between two errors. One error is ignoring every movement because fluctuation is normal. The other is treating every movement as a problem because it is visible. The regulatory frame avoids both. It asks whether movement is coordinated across time.

A single movement may be ordinary in isolation but meaningful if it repeats, extends, or layers with other constraints. A rise that resolves cleanly differs from a rise that remains prolonged. A decline that settles differs from a decline that triggers rebound. A fasting pattern that remains contained differs from one that becomes increasingly variable under stress or poor recovery.

Baseline, variability, and return are especially important to this framing. Baseline tendency describes where the system ordinarily starts and returns. Variability describes the movement around that tendency. Return describes whether movement resolves cleanly or requires increasing regulatory effort.

A system can move and remain stable if it returns coherently. A system can appear calm in isolated moments while gradually drifting upward in baseline. A system can produce readings that are not dramatic individually while movement becomes more frequent, more prolonged, or slower to settle. Stability depends on pattern, not one point.

Response, correction, and recovery form the operating rhythm of stability. The system responds when fuel enters, when tissues demand energy, when food is absent, when stress signals readiness, and when sleep-wake transitions occur. It corrects movement through uptake, storage, release, preservation, and signal adjustment. It recovers when those responses resolve and the system returns toward a workable range.

Overcorrection shows why response alone is not enough. A corrective signal can be necessary and still overshoot. A glucose-lowering response can move too far. A glucose-raising response can persist too long. Correction can produce counter-correction, rebound, and oscillation. Stability requires responses that resolve rather than create the next disturbance.

Constraint-aware stability completes the frame. Blood sugar regulation does not occur with unlimited margin. Chronic stress, poor sleep, aging, illness burden, low recovery capacity, reduced muscle buffer, baseline elevation, repeated volatility, and overcorrection all shape how much room the system has for clean adjustment.

Constraint does not mean failure. It means regulation is operating under limits. The same input, fasting interval, stress signal, sleep disruption, or activity demand can produce different movement depending on available margin. Stability is not perfection under unlimited conditions. It is coordination within real system limits.

Micromanagement misreads this reality by treating ordinary regulatory movement as something that must be immediately corrected or explained by one cause. A regulated system needs movement, adaptation, release, uptake, correction, and return. Over-isolating each number can make the larger pattern harder to see.

The final interpretive shift is from isolated cause to system state. Instead of treating a visible number as self-explanatory, the regulatory frame asks what layers were interacting: input, output, release, signaling, fasting state, stress load, sleep and recovery, demand, baseline tendency, variability, and constraint. The number becomes a point of observation, not a verdict.

The same shift applies to the idea of control. The question is not how to force a line into stillness. The deeper question is how regulation coordinates input, output, release, demand, recovery, and constraint over time. This is not a behavioral instruction. It is a change in interpretation.

The Stability Framing Mechanism closes the central argument by replacing blood sugar as a number with blood sugar as a regulated system. A reading matters because it belongs to the system. A rise matters because it has context. A decline matters because it reflects tissue handling. A baseline matters because it shows the ordinary return point. Variability matters because it shows containment and recovery across time.

Blood sugar stability means regulation remains coordinated enough for movement to stay contained, interpretable, and recoverable. It allows for input, fasting, stress, sleep disruption, activity demand, internal release, uptake, storage, correction, and return. It does not require perfection, stillness, or moral judgment.

This framing also keeps the book's central argument intact. Food matters, but food is not the whole system. Insulin matters, but insulin is not the whole system. Fasting matters, but fasting is not the whole system. Stress, sleep, activity, recovery, liver release, tissue uptake, baseline, variability, and constraint all matter because they belong to one regulatory field. Blood sugar stability is the pattern that emerges from that field over time.

The final point is not that blood sugar should be ignored or feared less through reassurance. The point is that it should be interpreted at the correct level. A number belongs to a pattern. A pattern belongs to regulation. Regulation belongs to a constrained system coordinating fuel availability across changing conditions.

Blood sugar is therefore best understood as a regulated expression of fuel availability across time. It is not a score, a test of discipline, a perfect line, or a single number to isolate from the system that produced it. Stability is coordinated regulation across time, not judgment, perfection, or control of one visible value.

About the Author

Nathan Reed writes about metabolic stability in systems exposed to load, variability, and time.

His work examines how biological capacity is shaped by energy availability, recovery architecture, sleep amplitude, muscle mass, environmental demand and workload. Rather than treating nutrition, fasting, sleep, and training as isolated tactics, he approaches them as interacting regulatory systems governed by margin, buffering, oscillatory coherence, and constraint dominance.

The Stability framework explores how physiological compression accumulates gradually and how proportional calibration preserves long-horizon resilience across decades. The objective is not peak optimization, but preservation of functional continuity under load.

Blood Sugar Stability is part of a broader metabolic stability ecosystem developed under Perennial Publishing, each volume addressing a distinct vector of biological durability.

The work is designed for readers who prefer structural clarity over motivational rhetoric and long-horizon coherence over short-term intensity.

The Metabolic Stability Series

Metabolic Stability – (Cornerstone Volume)

Fasting Fundamentals – (Foundational Volume)

Intermittent Fasting

Prolonged Fasting

Electrolytes

Insulin Stability

Glucose Stability

Metabolic Flexibility

Appetite Stability

Energy Stability

Blood Sugar Stability: ***How Glucose Regulation, Insulin Feedback, Stress, Sleep, and Fasting Shape Metabolic Health***

Future Titles Include:

Fat Loss Stability

The Vitality Series:

Sleep and Recovery

Strength and Aging

Hormones & Sexual Health

Part of a Broader Stability Framework

The Metabolic Stability Series is part of a larger stability ecosystem published by Perennial Publishing.

Related domains include:

Money Stability — structural durability in financial systems

Career Stability — positioning, load tolerance, and transition resilience

Mental Stability — cognitive steadiness under pressure and uncertainty

Emotional Stability — regulatory steadiness in environments that do not slow down

Foundations — low-fragility life architecture

Vitality — energy, strength, and biological function across time

Each domain approaches stability as a structural problem: capacity versus load, buffering versus shock, governance versus drift. Together, they form a unified framework for long-horizon durability across the major systems that shape human trajectory.

About Perennial Publishing

Perennial Publishing produces practical systems guides for building stability in an unstable world.

Our books explore the foundations of long-term resilience across health, finance, career, and everyday decision-making. Each title focuses on clear frameworks, durable principles, and practical strategies that help readers build lasting stability rather than short-term fixes.

The Perennial catalog includes series on metabolic health, financial stability, career systems, and personal consistency. While each book stands on its own, they share a common goal: helping individuals create durable systems that support a stable and sustainable life.

Made in United States
North Haven, CT
04 November 2026

21768650R00092